SOTHIS PRESS

Sothis Press aims to completely reimagine the public domain book with an emphasis on universal access to captivatingly designed print editions. We believe that technology will enable every single book ever published to be perpetually accessible in beautiful print form. Sothis is beauty in ubiquity.

www.sothis.press
1 Waterhouse Square, London, ECIN 2ST

Contributions to the Physiology and Pathology of the Circulation of the Blood

George Robinson

SOTHIS PRESS

ISBN 978-1-0368-0063-5

Contributions to the Physiology and Pathology of the Circulation of the Blood
is in the public domain.

This edition is published by
Sothis Press © 2023. The company
is registered in England and Wales.
The Company Number is 14900389.

ON THE

CIRCULATION OF THE BLOOD.

LONDON:
Printed by SPOTTISWOODE & Co.
New-street Square.

CONTRIBUTIONS

TO THE

PHYSIOLOGY AND PATHOLOGY

OF THE

CIRCULATION OF THE BLOOD.

BY

GEORGE ROBINSON, M.D.

LICENTIATE OF THE ROYAL COLLEGE OF PHYSICIANS OF LONDON;
JOINT LECTURER ON THE PRINCIPLES AND PRACTICE OF PHYSIC IN THE NEWCASTLE-ON-TYNE COLLEGE OF MEDICINE IN CONNECTION WITH THE UNIVERSITY OF DURHAM;
PHYSICIAN TO THE NEWCASTLE AND GATESHEAD DISPENSARIES; AND
PHYSICIAN TO, AND MEDICAL PROPRIETOR OF, BENSHAM ASYLUM, GATESHEAD.

LONDON:
LONGMAN, BROWN, GREEN, LONGMANS, & ROBERTS.
1857.

TO

THOMAS HODGKIN, M.D.

MEMBER OF THE SENATE OF THE UNIVERSITY OF LONDON,

AND

WILLIAM BOWMAN, F.R.S.

SURGEON TO KING'S COLLEGE AND THE ROYAL OPHTHALMIC HOSPITALS,

THE FOLLOWING PAGES ARE

Inscribed,

AS A SLIGHT TRIBUTE OF RESPECT FOR DISTINGUISHED
PROFESSIONAL ATTAINMENTS,

OF ESTEEM FOR EMINENT PRIVATE WORTH,

AND OF GRATITUDE FOR MANY ACTS OF KINDNESS
RENDERED TO THEIR

SINCERELY ATTACHED FRIEND,

GEORGE ROBINSON.

INTRODUCTORY REMARKS.

"DENIQUE in omni parte medicinæ, physiologicâ, pathologicâ, semeioticâ, therapeuticâ, cum quot problemata determinari possint ex hac datâ veritate et luce, quanta dubia solvi et quot obscura dilucidari, animo mecum reputo, campum invenio spatiosissimum, ubi longius percurrere et latius expatiari adeo possum, ut non solum in volumen excresceret, præter institutum meum, hoc opus, sed mihi forsan vita ad finem faciendum deficeret."*

"It must be confessed that the discovery of the circulation has not been followed by so great an advancement in the science of medicine as was naturally to have been expected from it. The reason of which is, that our theory has not yet advanced much in the knowledge which is naturally

* Harvey, "De Cordis et Sanguinis Motu." 1648.

founded upon this grand principle — *the circulation.* It has not yet explained the epicycles, as I may be allowed to call the partial systems, and various relations of parts, both fluid and solid, on which the anomalies of the body, the nature of diseases, and the operations of medicines must depend. Had Newton only discovered the general operation of gravity upon all matters, and barely hinted that the motion of the planets must depend upon it, philosophers had then understood the system of the world nearly as well as we do now the system of the body." *

A conviction of the truth of the opinions expressed in the preceding quotations, led me, many years since, to engage in an attempt to elucidate some points in the physiology of the circulation of the blood, and to apply that great principle more extensively to the illustration and explanation of pathological phenomena. For, since all experience shows us that the incessant and regular motion of the blood is, in the human body, the source and supporter of those secondary functions which collectively constitute Animal Life, it seems but natural to seek in its irregularities and disorders for

* An Epistle to the Rev. Dr. Hales, introductory to an Essay on the Blood. By Richard Davies, M.D. Bath, 1759.

a key to many of the morbid actions which have hitherto remained inexplicable. Why the study of the phenomena of the circulation, of the laws regulating it in health and disease, and of the contrivances by which its various effects are produced, has hitherto remained an almost untrodden field, is a question which I shall not now stop to discuss, and I allude to it only as an excuse for my own deficiencies.

It would have been more consonant to my own original intention, and perhaps have met with more general approval, had the matter contained in the following pages been systematically arranged. But as the preparation of a treatise at all worthy of the subject, one giving even an outline of the Physiology and Pathology of the Circulation of the Blood, would have involved the devotion of more time and thought than I can spare from the active duties of life; and as there are still some very important points connected with the views now submitted on which I believe it possible to throw much additional light, I am induced to be content at present with collecting a few papers from different periodicals and adding to them one or two more recent essays on the same subject.

I have altered nothing in the papers now reprinted, believing it to be due to myself and others to allow them to remain as published. But as the first is extracted from a little pamphlet on Bright's Disease of the Kidney, I have merely retained the passages bearing most directly on the subject of this publication.

Among the questions examined are the Mechanism of Absorption and Effusion, the Existence of an Extra-vascular Circulation, the Nature and Principles of Treatment of Inflammation and the Allied Disorders of the Circulation, and the Pathology of Albuminuria, Calcareous Degeneration, Epilepsy, Apoplexy, and some forms of Nervous Disorder. The following is the order in which they have been investigated.

Inflammation and the Allied Disorders of the Circulation of the Blood. (Page 124.)

6. On the Pathological changes occurring in certain Devitalised Tissues. (Page 246.)

7. On the peculiarities of the Cerebral Circulation, and their connection with the Pathology of Epilepsy and Apoplexy. (Page 257.)

8. On the Influence exercised in Health and Disease upon the Sensorial Functions of the Cerebro-Spinal Nerves by the state of the Circulation in the adjacent Blood-vessels. (Page 267.)

NEWCASTLE-ON-TYNE:
25, Eldon Square.
September 12th, 1857.

CONTRIBUTIONS

TO THE

PHYSIOLOGY AND PATHOLOGY

OF THE

CIRCULATION OF THE BLOOD.

ON THE MODE OF PRODUCTION OF

ALBUMINOUS URINE IN GRANULAR (BRIGHT'S) DISEASE OF THE KIDNEY.

[From an Inquiry into the Nature of Granular Disease of the Kidney, and its Mode of Action in producing Albuminous Urine. London: 1842.]

PERHAPS the most important, and certainly not the least difficult part of the subject, is the explanation of the peculiarities in the composition of the urine secreted in the different stages of this disease, comprising its albuminous impregnation and its low specific gravity.

It may be well, before entering on the exposition of the views which I have been led to adopt on this point, to mention briefly the various theories which have been advanced for the purpose of solving the difficulty caused by the unnatural existence of albumen in this secretion.

The one, perhaps most generally adopted, supposes that this effect is the result of a peculiar irritation of the kidney, induced by, or at least connected with, the granular deposit in that organ. No reason however is given why the same disordered state of the gland should not be produced by other diseases affecting it; and indeed the theory seems refuted by the fact of the proportion of albumen in the urine being often diminished in the advanced stages, when the granular deposit occupies most of the organ, and any irritability of the kidney, consequent on its presence, will be at a maximum. Whereas the contrary should occur were there any fixed relation between the proportion of albumen in the urine and the quantity of granular matter in the renal substance.

Another hypothesis, still more untenable, is that the albumen either supplies the place of urea, or is a transposition of its elements. This idea falls at once to the ground, as urea is known to be excreted up to the very last stage; and when death follows suppression of urine it is found in the blood and dropsical effusions: indeed its non-elimination seems incompatible with life. The quantity of it discharged from the system in the advanced stages of the disease is said to be less than in health; but when speaking of the causes of the low specific gravity of the urine a reason for this occurrence will be suggested which is simple, and adequate to its explanation.

Since studying this subject and arriving at the conclusions which I am about to relate, I find that the same hypothesis, as to the cause of albuminous urine, has been thrown out by others; but as it has not yet to my knowledge been supported by a close examination of all the cases in which albuminous urine has occurred, and has been advanced in a vague and undefined form, I trust that I may still be allowed to claim a share in whatever credit the fact of having first established a fixed and general rule for the explanation of the presence of albumen in the renal secretion may be considered to deserve.

Dr. Williamson, in the last number of the "Edinburgh Medical and Surgical Journal," mentions this hypothesis, viz. that albuminous urine is produced by congestion of the kidney, but he seems to consider it as occurring from a state of the lining membrane of the pelvis, analogous to that of the serous membranes in dropsy, or in other words from a disturbance of the balance between exhalation and absorption. As there is so much difference in the structure and function of mucous and serous membranes, the comparison, if I understood it correctly, does not seem a good one. The same gentleman also mentions a diseased condition of the blood, such as that existing in scurvy, as likely to cause albuminous or bloody urine; and the probability of such an occurrence should be borne in mind in investigating the cause of albuminuria in any particular case.

Having now stated all the theories that I know to have been advanced for the purpose of explaining the production of this peculiarity, I will next proceed to sketch the train of reasoning by which I was led to arrive at the discovery of a very simple rule for its explanation.

The first step to be taken is to have as clear a view as possible of the nature of the mechanism by which healthy secretion is performed. There are certain difficulties and mysteries attending this vital process which have not yet, and perhaps never will be, fully understood; but there are some facts now pretty universally admitted with respect to secretion in general, and that of the kidneys in particular, which I may be allowed briefly to enumerate.

1. All secreted fluids escape through the porous coats of the capillaries into the excretory ducts, or recipient cavities, where a free surface exists, and not from the open mouths of exhalent vessels as was formerly imagined.

2. The principles of which some, if not all, secretions are composed, exist previously in the mass of the circulating fluid; this is especially the case with the secretion of the kidneys, and hence their function would seem to be limited to the task of eliminating or selecting from the blood, during its passage through their capillaries, those substances, by the union of which healthy urine is constituted.

It is also probable that the structure of glands exerts some influence on the nature of the secreted products, otherwise the differences observed with regard to the length, situation, and minute arrangement of their constituent vessels and ducts would not have existed, for we never find nature to employ a complicated form of apparatus when a more simple one would answer the same end.

I would next direct attention to some circumstances connected with *albuminous* effusion, as a product of inflammation, and more particularly to the accompanying physical condition of the vessels through which it exudes.

When congestion is set up in the vessels of the cellular tissue of the body, which in health allow the escape of only a very fine vapour through their pores, we find an increased exudation, causing watery effusion, or œdema, to occur as the speedy consequence of the application of a slight obstructing cause to the circulation through them. If the congestion be greater, so as to be attended with the ordinary signs of inflammation, then albuminous effusion is observed to take place; and thus Muller says, "If a part, the subject of inflammation, has a free surface, whether there be a wound or not, an exudation of a coagulable fluid (the liquor sanguinis) takes place." The effect of a free surface in favouring effusion we see illustrated in the rapidity with which serous and albuminous infiltration of the loose cellular tissue of the scrotum follows inflammation, and the same remark will apply to the chemosis attending conjunctivitis.

When a ligature is tied round a limb so as slightly to obstruct the return of venous blood from it, at the end of a period, varying with circumstances, serous effusion into the cellular tissue or œdema is found to have taken place. In old and debilitated persons, from insufficient arterial impulse, and also from diminished contractile power of the capillaries, the same circumstance occurs spontaneously.

In the disease called phlegmasia dolens, or that in which there is a pale inelastic swelling of the leg, arising from the obstruction of the femoral vein by phlebitis, it may be presumed that the congestion of the capillaries has been sufficient to cause albuminous effusion into the cellular tissue.

In certain organs of the body, which are liable to sudden and great increase in the quantity of blood sent to them, nature seems to have taken precautions and made arrangements in their structure to prevent this effect of congestion from resulting.

Thus, in erectile tissue, the veins are large and numerous, and form either plexuses or cells, into which the excess of blood is received, and from which, when the inordinate action of the arteries has ceased, it gradually flows out,—albuminous effusion being also prevented by the dense fibrous tissue surrounding the vessels. In the spleen, a somewhat similar disposition occurs, probably for the same reason.

The differences observed in their natural and morbid secretions between the serous and mucous membranes are also worthy of consideration, as bearing in some measure on this point.

The structure of the former membranes is very dense, their vessels are so minute as not to admit the entrance of the red particles of the blood, and a fine vapour is the only transudation through their coats. When, from increased arterial action, a state of acute congestion is produced, it is evident that each vessel, being surrounded on all sides but one by the firm unyielding tissue of the membrane, can only relieve itself by effusion in that one direction, and on that point therefore the whole force of the distending pressure will act. The contractility of the capillaries is soon exhausted, and the impulse still continuing albuminous effusion takes place. In some instances the fluid thus poured out, though in considerable quantity, has contained so much fibrine, and retained so much of the vital property of the blood, as to coagulate spontaneously when removed from the body after death: in ordinary cases it is capable of organisation, and forms adhesions. When the inflammàtion is chronic, or the congestion less intense, the effusion proceeds more slowly, contains less albumen, and more nearly resembles the products of inflammation of the mucous membranes. These latter are looser in their texture, their vessels comparatively large and numerous, and the porous coats of the capillaries more lax, so that transudation takes place more readily through them. When an increased quantity of blood is determined to the vessels of a mucous tract, which had been previously in a healthy state, the immediate effect is a suppression of their secretion, from the capillaries contracting at first on the application of their stimulus. But as they soon begin to yield to the distending force, and become relaxed, the thinner portion of the contained blood escapes in the form of a copious watery discharge. In ordinary inflammation this discharge gradually diminishes in quantity and increases in its consistence, probably from its slower secretion and the evaporation or absorption of its more aqueous particles. We find this progress to convalescence to be hastened by the use of local and general stimulants of such moderate power as is best calculated to restore the tone of the capillaries. When the congestion is very intense, or when that part of the membrane affected is closely attached to bone or cartilage, so as more nearly to resemble the structure of serous membrane, then a more albuminous matter exudes and forms false membranes, as in inflammation of the larynx, trachea, or pharynx; but these are rarely organised, and the reason of this is not very obvious. Probably several circumstances unite in preventing its occurrence in mucous membranes; thus the effusion will be disturbed by the passage of various matters along the canal, its temperature will be thus affected, the secretion of mucus from any healthy part will also become mixed with it and prevent its close adaptation to the inflamed membrane, and the impulse of distension, or the compressing force applied to the vessels of the latter, may not be sufficient to cause organisation of the deposit, whilst all the opposite conditions to these may be shown to occur in inflamed serous membranes.

In procuring the direct union of divided parts, a certain amount of increased action is known to be necessary for the effusion of an organisable albumen, and in surgical practice these views as to the nature of the agency by which that effusion is effected have been long acted upon. In weak and debilitated subjects the surgeon endeavours to induce the adhesive process by giving stimulants so as to increase the force and frequency of the circulation, and thus cause the necessary degree of congestion in the adjacent vessels from which the effusion takes place: if the arteries of the part do not take on increased action, then no lymph is effused and union does not take place, and if that action is not continued a certain length of time, organisation of the effusion is arrested and suppuration results.

In chronic inflammation or passive congestion, as in indolent ulcers, in which the capillaries are relaxed and the arterial action is below the healthy standard, the secretion is thin and watery, but the flow of blood being increased, and an additional impulse given to that contained in the part by general and local stimulants, the effusion becomes more albuminous, healthy pus and granulations are formed, whilst the capillaries gradually begin to recover their tone on the application of their natural stimulus.

Many more facts might be brought forward in support of this view, but perhaps those I have mentioned are sufficiently numerous to justify me in saying, that *albuminous effusion* is always the consequence of a congested or distended state of the capillaries of the part, and that in a healthy condition of the blood the *proportion* of albumen in the effused fluid may be considered as commensurate with the *degree* of that congestion.

There are some circumstances which render it highly probable that the nutrition and growth of the different parts of the body are effected, in the first instance, by the effusion of albumen in a similar manner. Wherever active nutrition is going on, the arteries of the part are observed to carry more blood. This enlargement of the arteries will cause some distension and relaxation of the capillaries, as they cannot at once accommodate their calibre and contractility to the greater quantity of blood forced into them; effusion of a more or less albuminous nature will follow, and by its organisation the mass of the particular organ will be increased. In childhood, where growth and nutrition go on so rapidly, the size of the arteries is relatively greater than at any other period of life; and wherever the formative action proceeds with the greatest activity, there a disposition of the vessels favourable to congestion, and consequently to albuminous effusion, may be observed to exist.

In the impregnated uterus we have a still more striking example of the connexion which exists between a congested state of the vessels and the process of growth or nutrition. The spermatic and uterine arteries soon become enlarged and very tortuous, the corresponding veins accompanying them in their curves, *albuminous effusion* quickly takes place from the vessels lining the uterine cavity, it becomes organised, and the decidual membranes are formed. In the meantime a similar state of congestion has been produced in the capillaries of its muscular and cellular coats, albumen is there also effused, and when organised assumes the nature of these textures, and thus the whole organ is increased in size. The same arrangement of the vessels so essential to the growth of the uterus and to the nutrition of the fœtus continues during gestation, till parturition having taken place, the necessity for it ceases, and the arteries remitting their abnormal action the newly organised tissues become gradually absorbed. According to this view of the process, inflammation can only be considered as the extreme degree or improper application of a natural and healthy action; and hence the term as usually meant to signify a disease is not perhaps applicable to the processes of reparation or adhesion, and should only be used when speaking of those cases in which the congestion is either very acute, or occurs in parts where, or under circumstances when, its continuance is likely to disturb the nervous system and thus affect the health of the individual, or to prove injurious or inconvenient from the effects to which it may give rise.

But there are two instances of the appearance of albumen in secretions naturally not containing that principle, which bear still more directly on the subject under consideration.

In cows it is a well known fact that when the mammary vessels become distended from the increased determination of blood to them about the time of parturition, the fluid first secreted, termed colostrum, is scanty and bloody, and that it afterwards flows in greater quantity and not discoloured from blood, and is then so *highly albuminous* as to be used in domestic economy as a substitute for eggs, becoming a solid mass on boiling. Here the same explanation is available: the arteries acting with unusual power force a great quantity of blood into the minute capillaries of the gland, these become swollen and distended, and till they have time to accommodate themselves to their contents a variable degree of congestion, causing various kinds of effusion, is necessarily produced. At first it is so intense as to rupture some of the smaller vessels, and thus cause the presence of blood in the secretion; as these enlarge, it diminishes so much in degree as to be attended with only an albuminous exudation, the relative proportion of albumen present in the effused fluid gradually decreasing as the congestion is removed, till it finally ceases to be recognisable on the application of the same test (heat) for its detection.

Again, the saliva in health does not contain albumen, at least its quantity is not sufficient to affect the ordinary tests for its presence, but in that secreted during the congested state of the salivary glands, which attends mercurial action, it has been found always to exist; and here also, if the point were investigated, the proportion of albumen would doubtless be found to vary with the degree of that congestion.

From the consideration of all these circumstances, I would venture to propose the adoption of the following rule as adequate to the explanation of the cause of albuminous urine in nearly every case in which it may be observed to occur, viz.—

That the presence of albumen in the urine is produced by, and its proportional quantity is in a direct ratio to the degree of, congestion of the capillaries of the kidney, from whatsoever cause that congestion may arise.

Having now, I trust, satisfactorily proved that the only condition necessary for the exudation of albumen, and its subsequent appearance in any secretion, is a certain degree of congestion of the secreting gland, it only remains for me to show that such a state of the kidneys may exist in all those diseases which are attended with albuminous urine.

I need not again recapitulate any of the facts and arguments before advanced, to show that in acute nephritis a very high degree of congestion must naturally be present in the inflamed organ; but, taking this fact for granted, would next direct attention to the bloody and highly albuminous urine secreted in this disease, and to the corroboration which this fact, and the corresponding result obtained in the experiments hereafter mentioned, furnish in support of the correctness of the above rule, and more especially of that part of it which assumes the existence of a relation between the proportion of albumen in the urine and the degree of congestion in the kidney. It would seem that the intense degree of congestion accompanying acute glandular inflammation may also explain another effect of the latter, viz. the diminution or suppression of the secretion. For independently of its action in exhausting the nervous energy of the part and the healthy sensibility of the capillaries, it is evident from the anatomical structure of glands, and from the manner in which the capillaries surround the minute divisions of the excretory ducts, that when the former become much swollen from distension the pressure of their expansion must necessarily tend to compress and approximate the walls of, and hence obliterate the cavity naturally existing in the latter, so that the free surface essential for secretion no longer occurs; whence in the case of the kidneys, retention of urea in the blood and the not unfrequent occurrence of death as the termination of one of the forms of coma described by Dr. Addison.

In chronic nephritis a minor degree of congestion exists, for the blood does not enter the renal arteries with so powerful an impulse or in such large quantity as in acute inflammation; and hence in the former the relative quantity of albumen in the urine is less. Other causes probably tend also to the same end; for, in addition to the heart participating in the general debility, as shown by the decreased power and activity of the circulation, the blood as the disease advances contains less albumen than in health; and being largely composed of water its tenuity favours transudation, and its more aqueous portion escapes in the form of urine of a low specific gravity. When, from the operation of any accidental cause, there is an unusual determination to the kidneys, the congestion will naturally be for the time increased, and as an immediate consequence, more albumen will be effused into the urine. But on the other hand, if no unnatural excitement, causing increased action of the renal vessels, take place for a length of time, the latter will become accommodated to their contents, and the albumen thus lost to the system may be reduced to a very minute quantity, or altogether cease, but will be immediately reproduced on the recurrence of any increase of vascularity and congestion. Both these alternations have been observed in the progress of disease, and afford additional proofs of the truth of the above theory.

When chronic inflammation causes the deposit of a solid matter in the vascular tissue of the organ, a state of more or less congestion must evidently be produced in the remainder. For this deposit occupies the place of blood-vessels, compresses those contiguous to it, and ultimately causes their destruction, while, as the renal arteries bring in as much blood as when all the vessels of the gland existed, it follows that more than usual must be distributed to the remaining ones; and as the number of those still pervious is gradually reduced by the obliteration of fresh vessels, a degree of engorgement of them must occur to some extent. It is from the slow and gradual manner in which the deposition generally takes place that the quantity of albumen effused is so small in proportion to the extent of vascular tissue destroyed, as the remaining vessels have had time to enlarge; but when the morbid action goes on most rapidly, the proportion of albumen in the urine will be greater, and in the most insidious cases it will be very minute.

Applying this reasoning not only to the more regular form of chronic inflammation, or that in which the kidneys are granular or mottled, but to all kinds of morbid deposit in these organs, we shall see how far they admit of a similar explanation. Cases of albuminous urine from other causes have been met with—by Solon in dropsy and obliteration of the cortical portion by cysts: by Rayer in three cases, one of hæmaturia with cancer and calculus in the kidney, another of true tubercular disease of it, and the third of inflammation of that organ and the bladder; by Christison in cerebriform disease; and by Syme in strumous disease.

There is another class of cases in which, from various causes, the circulation through the abdominal and renal veins becomes more or less obstructed, and thus sometimes spontaneously, perhaps more frequently from the conjoined effect of accidental determination to the kidneys, a sufficient degree of congestion of these organs is produced to cause the temporary appearance of albumen in the urine. Thus it has been observed in cases of peritonitis (probably affecting chiefly that portion adjacent to the kidneys) by Nystel and others; in pregnancy by Rayer; during the crisis of fever, certain cutaneous affections, and some inflammatory diseases (particularly pneumonia), by Solon; in hypertrophy of the heart, with valvular obstruction, by M. Fourget; in chronic inflammation of the liver by Graves; in phthisis, sometimes slightly in diabetic urine, and in a few other cases, in all of which, either from suspension of the cutaneous function and consequent increased action of the kidneys, or from a direct obstruction to the venous circulation in which the renal veins participated, some degree of congestion in these organs may naturally be supposed to have existed.

It is now necessary for me to state the exceptions to the above rule, which are chiefly of importance from their interfering with, and in some measure diminishing, the value which might otherwise be attached to albuminous urine as a test of the presence, and even of the degree of renal congestion. They may be briefly stated to be comprised in those cases in which pus or other albuminous matter is suspended in the urine from inflammation of some part of the genito-urinary mucous membrane. Thus it has been found more or less albuminous in cases of old and severe stricture, in a bladder inflamed and irritated by a calculus, during the passage of a calculus down the ureter, and would probably present the same character if examined in the acute stage of gonorrhœa; but it must also be remembered that these affections will each ultimately tend to produce renal congestion and irritation, so that in old cases it will sometimes be a doubtful point to determine whether the albumen is derived from the inflamed mucous membrane or from the kidney.

A diseased condition or unnatural fluidity or tenuity of the blood, as in scurvy, or that peculiar condition of the vessels which induces excessive hæmorrhage from slight causes, and which has been found hereditary in some instances, may each cause the presence of albumen or blood in the urine.

Considerable importance has been attached to the low specific gravity of the urine, as characteristic of granular disease: in the acute form its density is at least equal to that of health, and it is only in the advanced stages of the chronic form that the proportion of solids contained in it is materially reduced. Some relative deficiency may be referrible to the fact of the quantity of water in which they are suspended being increased, but it would appear established that there is a decided falling off in the gross amount of solids discharged from the system, and this may be explained in the following manner. Urea is found in the blood: it would seem to be the product of a species of decomposition of animal matter going on during the circulation of that fluid, the quantity of it excreted from the system being greatest after the consumption of azotised food, and commensurate with the proportion of animal principles existing in the blood. Now, during the progress of chronic nephritis it has been shown that the blood becomes impoverished, the albumen escaping from it in the urine being replaced by water, and the debility being still further increased from the impediment to nutrition occasioned by the frequent complication of vomiting and diarrhœa.

The substitution of water for the important principle, albumen, must necessarily diminish the quantity of those azotised matters formed in the blood by the decomposition or deterioration of its more animalised portion, and hence the deficiency of urea and the lithates in this disease. Viewed in this light, the low specific gravity of the urine cannot be considered as indicating more than an impoverished condition of the blood, which state we know may also occur in many other diseases, and hence any value which might otherwise attach to this symptom as diagnostic of this particular affection must be rendered doubtful till future experiments shall decide as to whether a similar state of the urine does not accompany the same condition of the blood in every disease in which the latter is present, as after long continued suppurative or other albuminous discharges.

From reflecting on the great obstruction to the circulation through the minute vessels of an inflamed part, I was led to imagine, that by preventing the return of blood from the kidney in one of the lower animals, and taking care not to injure the artery in the experiment, a condition of the organ, similar to that present in acute nephritis, would be produced, which might throw some light on those points in which the latter disease differed from the acute stage of granular kidney. Accordingly I cut down to and exposed one kidney in a rabbit and tied the renal vein, returning the organ immediately into its natural position with the artery uninjured. The animal died about fifteen hours afterwards, and on examination the kidney in question was the only organ found affected; it was intensely congested and very much enlarged, being nearly twice the bulk and weight of the healthy organ; of a dark red or blackish colour, in some places soft and easily torn, and the granular appearance on its surface more distinct than natural, as if from enlargement of the granules. On making a section it was throughout intensely gorged with blood, which seemed infiltrated into the cellular tissue of the organ: *there was a little bloody urine in the bladder which contained two or three minute coagula, and became nearly a solid mass on applying heat.* This experiment was repeated with precisely the same results as to the condition of the kidney, but from the ureter having been divided and tied, the urine secreted could not be examined. Perhaps the value of any conclusions drawn from these facts is increased from the circumstance of M. Rayer and Dr. Osborne having found fibrinous clots filling the renal veins in those who had died in the acute stage, an occurrence which shows that a very imperfect and retarded, if not a completely obstructed, circulation through those vessels had existed during life.

The granular appearance of the exterior was also more distinct in the congested kidney, arising from the distension of the granules naturally existing there.

Such are the morbid appearances of the most acute form when it has proved rapidly fatal; but it is a point of some importance to learn the nature of the changes which take place in cases where the patients are not so rapidly cut off by the disease.

There is an interesting case of acute idiopathic nephritis related by Mr. Snow, in a late number of the American Journal of Medical Sciences: the patient died at the end of nine days, the secretion of urine during that time having been entirely suppressed, and symptoms of poisoning from the retention of urea in the blood having preceded death. On examination, the left kidney was atrophied, and on inquiry it was ascertained, that several years before she had an attack of some nephritic disease, which, from the symptoms mentioned by her friends, was probably of the same nature as that which proved fatal. In the recently inflamed organ, the cortical portion to about half its extent was opaque, whitish, and seemed infiltrated with lymph, a little serum oozing out, but no pus; there was a white deposit in diffused patches, and a few small scattered spots over the whole cortical part; the tissues of the organ were rather fluid and friable; there was a minute quantity of dirty, dark, brownish urine.

These appearances correspond very closely with those observed in a rabbit in which I exposed the kidney and passed a thread under the renal vein, allowing it to remain there with the view of inducing slow obliteration of that vessel and a simultaneous congestion of the kidney. It died nine days afterwards, and on examination, the kidney operated on was, if anything, rather smaller than natural; its surface seemed to want the smooth convexity of the healthy organ, as though its bulk had been recently diminished; on the exterior, and diffused through the substance of the cortical tissue, were irregular white patches of lymph, and the remains of several ecchymoses, the colouring matter of which had been partly absorbed. The other kidney was considerably congested, and *the urine in the bladder moderately but distinctly albuminous,* both heat and nitric acid being applied.

These may be looked upon as the appearances which would generally result in cases where the inflammation has been very acute, and the patient has lived long enough for absorption to have diminished the bulk of the congested organ, constituting as it were the transition stage between the enlarged and engorged state of the kidney on the one hand, and its diminution and atrophy on the other. Were the obstruction to the circulation through the kidney and the consequent accumulation of blood in its vessels less intense in degree but longer-continued, then the increased size of the organ would be more permanent, and this would seem to occur in cases in which chronic nephritis has commenced as the primary disease; whilst atrophy and diminution, as in the left kidney of the case just quoted, seems more rapidly to follow acute congestion. And the reason of this is tolerably evident; for the obstruction to the circulation being more complete in acute inflammation, coagulation takes place more quickly in the minute vessels of the part, which are thus, to a certain extent, obliterated and rendered incapable of receiving the fresh arterial blood necessary for nutrition; whilst in chronic inflammation the coagulation of the blood in the relaxed capillaries goes on very slowly; and it is, therefore, evident that the filling up or occupation of the *dilated* capillaries by fibrinous coagula must then necessarily cause an increase in the bulk of any organ which is mainly composed of these vessels.

RESEARCHES

INTO THE CONNECTION EXISTING BETWEEN

AN UNNATURAL DEGREE OF COMPRESSION OF THE BLOOD CONTAINED IN THE RENAL VESSELS,

AND

THE PRESENCE OF CERTAIN ABNORMAL MATTERS IN THE URINE.

[From the twenty sixth volume of the MEDICO-CHIRURGICAL TRANSACTIONS, published by the Royal Medical and Chirurgical Society of London. Communicated by MARSHALL HALL, M.D., F.R.S., &c. Read February 14th, 1843.]

HAVING undertaken some experiments with the view of determining the precise cause of the appearance of albumen in the urine, I found that not only liquid albumen and blood, but coagulating lymph or fibrine also escaped into the urinary passages as the consequence of an obstruction to the return of blood through the renal vein. As the unnatural compression of the blood in the renal vessels, thus artificially produced, gave rise to phenomena identical with those constituting the primary effects of inflammation, and as the kidney seemed to present greater facilities for an experimental investigation of that important subject than any other organ of the body, I was induced to extend my observations, and to attempt certain modifications of the experiment. The facts thus obtained will, I think, enable us to explain, with more precision than has hitherto been attempted, the true reason of the variable nature of the effusion in different instances: and as this involves physiological and pathological points of some importance, the question may not be deemed unworthy of the consideration of the Society.

As a full description of each experiment must necessarily involve much repetition, and might, therefore, tend to weary and distract the attention, I shall in this place content myself with relating those general results which bear directly on the main object of this communication, leaving the particulars of each experiment to be more minutely described in the appendix to these remarks. With the exception of the first, all these experiments were performed on the kidneys of rabbits. The animals employed varied much in age, size, and condition; and as the strength of the system exerted a very material influence in modifying the nature of the effusion, each experiment must be considered by itself, in order to arrive at a strictly accurate conclusion.

My reasons for selecting the kidney were the following:—

This organ can be readily and quickly exposed in the lower animals, and its artery, vein, and duct, (which constitute almost the sole bonds of union between it and the rest of the body,) may be separately secured by ligature; so that we not only have the circulation through the gland entirely under our command, but are, at the same time, enabled to isolate and confine the secretion, and thus prevent the possibility of error in examining the composition of the latter. Moreover, the recent discoveries of my friend Mr. Bowman, by clearing away the mystery which had previously surrounded the Malphigian bodies, have made us well acquainted with the minute anatomy of the kidney, and have thereby enabled us more clearly to understand the mechanism of the process.

Having obtained all that I expected from obstructing the return of blood through the renal vein, I was anxious to ascertain the effect of directing, with different degrees of rapidity, an increased flow of blood to the vessels of an organ previously healthy; the passage of this blood being unimpeded by any artificial obstacle, and the organ itself being untouched. After some unsatisfactory trials, I at length obtained results precisely similar to those met with in the former series after venous obstruction.

Although the same general effects were produced in all the experiments, it will be more advantageous to consider them as arranged under two divisions.

The first, containing twenty experiments, in all of which some artificial impediment obstructed the flow of blood through the vein.

The second, comprising fourteen experiments, in which an increased determination of blood was directed to one or both kidneys, without any artificial obstacle being opposed to its free return.

After the experiments on the kidneys were performed, it occurred to me, that the observation of the effects of venous obstruction in the vessels of a frog's foot might serve to illustrate the action of the same cause in the former cases.

Accordingly, the hinder extremity of a frog was so included within two ligatures that the artery and bone were the only parts left free. There was some slight oozing of serous fluid from the wound in the ham, and the limb below the ligature speedily became red and swollen. On looking at the vessels in the web with a moderate magnifying power, the veins were seen to be much enlarged, and, as it were, prolonged into the capillaries in consequence of the accumulation of blood in, and distension of, the latter.

At first sight, the blood appeared to have lost all motion; but on examining more attentively, some small arteries were observed in the act of pouring in fresh blood, the impulse of which propelled onwards the column in the veins at each contraction of the heart. During the cessation of that action a retrograde movement occurred, the two alternate actions causing an oscillation of the contained blood.

At the end of half an hour the globules had begun to cohere, and formed by their union irregular masses and cylindrical columns, which moved to and fro synchronously with the contraction and relaxation of the ventricle; the former motion being evidently produced by the momentum of the arterial blood, the latter resulting from the resiliency of the elastic tissues.

At the end of seven hours the blood was completely stagnant in all the vessels.

At some points slight extravasation had apparently taken place, for the red outline of the vessels was irregular and ragged. In other places the red line marking their breadth was uniform and even; but a white line of opacity (not unlike that caused in transparent tissues by the effusion of lymph) was situated externally to it.

Various stimulants were then applied to the web without producing any distinct effect either on the vessels or on the blood which they contained. The limb never recovered its vitality, and subsequently underwent the various changes of mortification.

As these effects were such as might have been expected from previous reasoning, and as they were precisely analogous to those which I presumed to occur in the minute vessels of the kidney during the existence of an obstruction to the circulation of the blood through them, I did not think it necessary to repeat the observation.

Class I.

ILLUSTRATING THE EFFECTS OF VENOUS OBSTRUCTION.

A.—The ligature around the renal vein being tightly applied, and no hæmorrhage occurring from any of its branches.

Number of Experiments.	Interval between the application of ligature and death of the animal.	Composition of the urine as regards the presence in it of albumen, lymph, or blood.
1	10 minutes.	Slightly albuminous.
2	30 minutes.	Ditto. ditto.
3	30 minutes.	No urine in bladder; ureter not examined.
4	10 minutes.	Highly albuminous.
5	6 minutes.	Very highly albuminous, and some slight appearance of fibrine.
6	3½ minutes.	Bloody.
7	1 hour.	Ditto.

These experiments alone suffice to show that the same kind of effusion does not necessarily and constantly result from the existence of the same degree of obstruction. It will be evident that this latter constitutes but one of the conditions required to cause the exudation of the more viscid portion of the blood through the coats of its containing vessels. A certain amount of impulse of the arterial blood must always co-exist and co-operate with the obstruction, before that species of effusion can take place. The activity of this force will of course be proportioned to the rapidity and vigour of the ventricular contractions; and it is to the varied power of the heart's action, at the moment of applying the ligature, that I ascribe the different results met with in the above experiments. I have throughout invariably observed that the effects of an intense degree of compression were chiefly to be expected in those instances where the animal seemed to recover most speedily from the shock of the operation.

B.—The obstruction of the renal vein being either incomplete or gradually effected.

In 6 cases some venous hæmorrhage occurred from accidental or intentional laceration of the vein or its branches.

In 2, the coats of the vessel were raised by a forceps, and a ligature so applied as to include only half the vein; leaving it at the moment pervious, though of diminished calibre.

In 4, a thread was passed around the vein, and so tied as to enclose the latter within a loose loop; the vessel itself not being compressed by the ligature.

—
12

The results will be most readily understood by a glance at the subjoined Table:

No. of each experiment as related in the Appendix.	Interval between the application of obstruction and death of the animal.	Composition of urine.
1	1 hour.	Slightly albuminous.
2	30 minutes.	Highly albuminous.
3	7 minutes.	Slightly albuminous.
4	1 hour.	A mass of lymph in the bladder.
5	1 hour.	Blood and fibrine.
6	1 hour.	Lymph and blood.
7	40 minutes.	Bloody.
8	$4\frac{1}{2}$ days.	Urine muddy and faintly albuminous.
9	18 hours.	Bloody.
10	1 hour.	Bloody.
11	24 hours. (?)	Moderately albuminous.
12	$2\frac{1}{2}$ days.	Reddened by blood, and highly albuminous.

The lymph found in the bladder, in one of these experiments (No. 4), was beautifully clear and pellucid. It was semi-fluid when first examined, but coagulated more firmly on exposure to the air.

I am not aware that any other instance is recorded of the effusion of coagulating lymph, as the consequence of simple compression of the blood from venous obstruction. The quantity was so considerable, in this case, and the manifestation of its peculiar properties so decided, that there was not the least room for doubt. The physical condition of the blood in the vessels of this kidney must have been that of a fluid subjected to a continued moderate pressure: for, in consequence of a slight laceration of the vein, the blood could not be compressed beyond a certain degree, as it would then tend to ooze through the lateral opening. I have not succeeded in obtaining so much lymph in any subsequent experiment. It must ever be a very difficult point so to adjust the obstruction to the amount of impulse of the arterial blood as to maintain the requisite degree of compression, and no more, for a sufficient length of time. The two succeeding experiments confirm the accuracy of the explanation just given: for in them the vein, being first tied tightly, was then punctured on the renal side of the ligature, so that a small jet of blood escaped. The organ being returned while in this condition, and the urine examined, at the end of an hour, both fibrinous and bloody coagula were found suspended in it. I think it not improbable that the blood, in these instances, escaped during the short interval that elapsed between the application of the ligature, and the puncture of the vein. For it will be remembered that, in a former case, blood was found in the urine at the end of three minutes and a half after the obstruction took place.

Three of the above experiments (viz., the 8th, 11th, and 12th) are related, not only for the illustration they afford of the general principle here advocated, but from their tending to throw light upon the changes which these engorged organs would subsequently undergo. The circumstance of blood and albumen being present in the urine at so late a period as the third or fourth day after the operation, may be partially explained by the slow progress of bloody or fibrinous coagula along the ureter. At the same time, I think it is possible that some albumen may have been derived from the other kidney, in consequence of the increased determination to that organ. I cannot help thinking that the morbid appearances which these three engorged kidneys presented, viz. the formation of an exterior membrane or cyst, the appearance of white spots on the external surface of the organ, as in Experiment 12, and the more extensive disintegration met with in Experiment 8, were but the first of a series of changes which would finally have terminated in the softening down of the whole organ, and its conversion into a puriform mass. And it seems by no means improbable that when abscess of the kidney follows acute nephritis in the human subject, the formation of a bag of pus (as met with in *post mortem* examinations) takes place in a similar manner, and is preceded by similar changes. An extended investigation of the changes which kidneys thus treated would finally undergo could not fail to throw important light on some of the secondary effects of inflammation.

I shall now pass on to the second class of experiments, or those intended to illustrate the effects of an increased determination of blood to the vessels of a part previously healthy.

It occurred to me, that if an increased flow of blood could be suddenly directed through any particular artery, the contractility of the smaller vessels would resist the rapid dilatation necessary for the free passage of the augmented quantity of fluid, and thus give rise to some obstruction. If any obstruction did take place, then both the conditions required to produce undue compression of the blood would co-exist, and some of its effects should be perceptible in the urine.

Class II.

A.—I first attempted to accomplish this end in the case of the renal artery by removing one kidney, thinking that the physiological determination to the other might suffice. I repeated the experiment five times, chiefly in young and weak animals. The only constant result observed was a progressive increase in the weight of the remaining kidney. In one instance there were some slight traces of albumen in the urine.

B.—I then, in two small weak animals, tied the abdominal aorta below the origin of the renal arteries. In one instance the urine was slightly albuminous.

C.—As I did not by these measures, used singly, obtain very satisfactory results, I then wished to ascertain whether the simultaneous performance of both operations *in animals of greater strength*, would not, by the conjoint influence of the physical and physiological determination of blood to the remaining kidney, induce the presence of albuminous matters in its secretion. I performed seven experiments. The three first did not succeed; but a glance at the particulars of each, as given in the Appendix, will, I think, suggest a satisfactory explanation of their failure. And any uncertainty which these negative results may have created as to the truth of the principle sought to be established in this part of the memoir, must be in a great measure removed by a careful perusal of the four last experiments. Thus, in—

	The animal living	
Exp. 4.	18 hours . . .	The urine contained blood, and the liquid portion albumen.
5.	About 2 days. .	It was highly albuminous.
6.	$3\frac{1}{2}$ hours . . .	A coagulum of blood, another of fibrine, and was highly albuminous.
7.	2 hours.	Blood and albumen.

In removing the left kidney, care was taken to secure the ureter as well as the blood-vessels. That these albuminous matters were derived from the right kidney, is proved beyond a doubt, by the existence of ecchymoses in its substance and on its surface in two instances, (Exp. 4 and 7,) by the increase of its weight, as seen in Exp. 6 and 7, and by the fact of the morbid products being detected in the right ureter in Exp. 6.

By selecting strong full-blooded animals, the repetition of this experiment would doubtless yield results precisely similar to those just detailed. I think the experiments related in the first division of this class, though yielding but negative evidence in support of the main point of this inquiry, are not altogether undeserving of consideration, and may be advantageously contrasted with the four last of the third division. For we learn from the former that a gradually increased quantity of blood may be directed to the vessels of a part without occasioning any material obstruction and compression of that fluid. While the concluding experiments show clearly that if the quantity determined to any particular set of vessels be considerably and *suddenly* increased, then some of the ordinary effects of undue compression of the blood will be produced.

Having now mentioned concisely the general results obtained, I may be allowed to allude again for a moment to those two conditions by which the compression of the blood in its vessels is produced and regulated.

This compression is altogether dependent upon

the co-existence and co-operation of two essential causes, each of which will, in different individuals, vary much in its amount of activity or degree of completeness.

The momentum of the arterial blood arising from the contractions of the ventricle constitutes the active force from the operation of which the compression takes place. But as a counter resistance is required before an intense degree of the latter state can occur, it is only when some extraordinary obstruction to the free passage of the blood *through the smaller vessels* exists that the effects of an undue compression of that fluid are perceptible.

It follows, therefore, that the momentum being equal in a number of cases, the intensity of the compression of the blood will be proportioned to the completeness of the obstruction: and, on the other hand, the impediment or obstruction being equally complete, the degree of compression will then be commensurate with the amount of the momentum.

The whole of the preceding experiments, if carefully considered, will, I think, support this statement.

They also prove—

1. That simple compression of the blood in its smaller vessels will, in a direct ratio to the degree of intensity of that compression, cause the exudation of an albuminous fluid, of coagulating lymph, or the extravasation of blood. Its immediate effects, therefore, precisely resemble those of inflammation: and as it is well ascertained that both the essential causes

of undue compression (viz. an obstruction or impediment to the flow of blood through the vessels of the inflamed part, and excessive action of the heart,) co-exist in that disease, it seems but reasonable to infer that the primary effects of inflammation, being identical with those of undue compression of the blood, are the mere consequences of that physical cause.

2. That there is no relation between the compositiou of the effused matters and the extent of the dilatation of the coats of the vessels, as measured by the quantity of blood they contain. To establish this point more clearly, I subjoin a short Table, exhibiting the relative weights of the healthy and engorged organs, and the nature of the effusion.

Order of the Experiments in the Appendix.	Weight of healthy kidney.	Weight of engorged kidney.	Relative Weights.	Condition of the urine.
Class 1.	grs.	grs.		
A. Exp. 1st.	20	40	1–2.	Faintly albuminous.
— 4th.	35	70	1–2.	Highly albuminous.
— 5th.	25	50	1–2.	Highly albuminous.
— 6th.	60	90	1–1.50	Bloody.
— 7th.	98	175	1–1.78	Bloody.
B. — 1st.	40	84	1–2.10	Slightly albuminous.
— 2nd.	50	150	1–3.	Highly albuminous.
— 4th.	100	130	1–1.30	A mass of lymph.
— 5th.	50	90	1–1.80	Bloody; with a fibrinous coagulum.
— 7th.	35	68	1–1.94	Bloody.
— 9th.	64	182	1–2.84	Bloody.
— 10th.	90	170	1–1.88	Bloody.

In conclusion, I may again repeat my opinion, that the process of the effusion of albumen and lymph through the coats of the vessels of the living body is dependent on, and regulated by, the degree of the compression of the blood contained within those vessels.

My chief object in undertaking this investigation was to endeavour to extend the application of ordinary physical laws to the explanation of some of the morbid and healthy phenomena of the animal body: for it seemed to me that if a few simple general principles could be established, we might then hope to understand more clearly the true nature of disease, and perhaps ultimately be enabled to treat it with greater success.

EXPERIMENTS ON THE KIDNEY.*

Class I.

ILLUSTRATING THE EFFECTS OF VENOUS OBSTRUCTION.

A.—The closure of the renal vein by ligature being immediate and complete.

Exp. 1. The left renal vein of a young weak rabbit was tied, and the animal killed at the end of ten minutes. The bladder was distended with urine, which, when tested by nitric acid and heat, presented

* Six of the experiments on venous obstruction were published in the Medical Gazette of June 1842; but as they serve to render the series more complete, and as the weight of the healthy and engorged kidneys was carefully ascertained, I have been induced to recapitulate them.

permanent flakes. The right kidney weighed 20 grs.; the left 40 grs.

Exp. 2. The same operation was performed on a rabbit of similar size and condition, which was killed at the end of half an hour. A smaller quantity of urine was found in the bladder, which, when tested by the same re-agents presented a more distinct flakiness. Weight of the right kidney, 26 grs.; of the left, 51 grs.

Exp. 3. A small weak animal was killed at the end of half an hour after ligature of the left renal vein. There was no urine in the bladder; the ureter was not examined. The right kidney weighed 26 grs.; the left, 50 grs.

Exp. 4. An animal of middle size, and in moderate condition, was killed ten minutes after ligature of the vein. There was about a drachm of urine in the bladder, which was highly albuminous. The right kidney weighed 35 grs.; the left 70 grs.

Exp. 5. The left vein and ureter being tied, in a young healthy rabbit, the animal was killed at the end of six minutes. The ureter being first carefully wiped, and then divided, the urine contained in it was allowed to drop on a watch-glass, and on being tested with nitric acid, it formed a solid clot. There was a slight appearance of coagulated lymph in the pelvis of the kidney, and a more copious effusion was found beneath its lining membrane. The bladder contained a drachm of urine, which was not albuminous. The right kidney weighed 25 grs.; the left 50 grs.

Exp. 6. The left renal vein of a middle-sized

healthy animal was tied, then the ureter, and exactly three minutes and a half after the ligature of the vein the artery was secured, and the organ removed. The ureter contained bloody urine. The right kidney was then removed: it weighed 60 grs.; the left 90 grs. The animal died towards the end of the second day, having previously manifested marked comatose symptoms. No morbid appearances worthy of mention were found.

Exp. 7. In a full grown, strong rabbit, the abdominal aorta was exposed by an incision on the left side of the spine, and seized by a powerful spring forceps. The hinder extremities were immediately paralysed. The blades of the forceps, the extremities of which were notched, were then separated and withdrawn; but, in taking this step, the coats of the artery became twisted and torn, and considerable hæmorrhage ensued. This was, however, arrested in a few minutes by compression of the trunk above. The left kidney was then drawn out through the same opening, its vein and ureter tied, and the organ returned. The animal seemed at first faint from the loss of blood, but gradually recovered; it was killed at the end of an hour; the paraplegia continuing unchanged till death. The left kidney was much engorged, and presented on its surface several spots of ecchymosis; it weighed 175 grs.; the right kidney, 98 grs. The left ureter contained a coagulum of blood, and above it some muddy brownish fluid, which, on exposure to the air, assumed a bright red tint. The bladder contained nearly two drachms of urine, which was natural in its appearance; and on being examined, contained no albumen, a few drops of nitric acid rendering it quite clear. The aorta had been torn rather more than two-thirds across; its compression, by the infiltration of the surrounding cellular tissue with a considerable quantity of blood, probably prevented the return of hæmorrhage by obliterating the vessel at that point.

B.—The canal of the renal vein being either partially or slowly obstructed.

Exp. 1. The animal was of middle size, but in poor condition. In tying the vein there was some hæmorrhage from a lateral branch. The animal had previously met with a slight accident, and seemed faint at the time; it was killed at the end of an hour, and the urine in the bladder was slightly but distinctly albuminous. The right kidney weighed 40 grs.; the left, 84 grs.

Exp. 2. In passing a ligature round the vein of a rabbit of middle size, and in moderate condition, the coats of the vessel were torn, and some hæmorrhage occurred, which was soon arrested by compression; it was killed at the end of half an hour. The bladder contained two drachms of urine which was highly albuminous. The right kidney weighed 50 grs.; the left, 150 grs.

Exp. 3. The left renal vein of a middle-sized weak rabbit was exposed, compressed for a few minutes, and then slightly torn, so as to allow a little blood to escape. The vessel was then securely tied, and the animal killed seven minutes after the application of the ligature. The urine in the bladder was very slightly albuminous. On dividing the left kidney, the lining membrane of the pelvis was rendered prominent by the deposition beneath, or external to it, of a quantity of clear lymph in which the larger branches of the vein were imbedded. There was no appearance of lymph in the cavity of the pelvis. The right kidney weighed 42 grs.; the left, 73 grs.

Exp. 4. In tying the vein of a strong full-grown rabbit, the coats of the vessel were slightly lacerated, so that a little blood continued to ooze out by the side of the ligature. In this state the organ was returned, and the animal killed at the end of an hour. Some urine had escaped through the urethra; but on laying open the bladder, it was found to contain a scruple, by weight, of clear pellucid lymph, which was semi-fluid when first examined, but coagulated more firmly on exposure to the air. The right kidney weighed 100 grs.; the left 130 grs.

Exp. 5. A middle-sized animal, in tolerable condition. The left renal vein was tied, and then punctured with a fine needle on the renal side of the ligature, so that some blood escaped in a fine jet. The organ was then returned within the walls of the abdomen, and the animal killed at the end of an hour. The bladder contained about two drachms of bloody urine, which held suspended in it a coagulum of fibrine. This latter was reddened only at one point; the rest of it being unstained by blood. The pelvis of the kidney also contained a small quantity of lymph: this organ weighed 90 grs.; the weight of the right one being 50 grs.

Exp. 6. The left renal vein of a small healthy animal was tied, and then lacerated on the renal side of the ligature. While bleeding freely, the organ was returned, and the animal killed at the end of an hour. The urine in the bladder was not albuminous; but the upper part of the ureter contained a column of lymph, which, at its lower end, was slightly tinged with blood. The left kidney was considerably enlarged, but the precise weight was not taken.

Exp. 7. In a young healthy rabbit the coats of the left vein were pinched up by a forceps, and so tied that the calibre of the venous canal would be considerably diminished. The animal was killed at the end of forty minutes. The bladder contained about a drachm of urine, which was not albuminous; but on further examination, the reason of this was apparent; for the left ureter was found completely obstructed by a coagulum of blood, behind which a quantity of bloody urine had accumulated. Some lymph had also been effused beneath the lining membrane of the pelvis. The right kidney weighed 35 grs.; the left, 68 grs.

Exp. 8. The left kidney being exposed in a healthy young rabbit, the coats of the vein were pinched up by a forceps, and so tied as materially to diminish the calibre of, without completely obstructing, the venous canal. The organ was then returned, and the animal killed at the end of four and a half days. The bladder contained a little muddy urine, which was faintly albuminous. The tubular portion of the right kidney was somewhat redder than usual. The left kidney was found enclosed within a perfect cyst of considerable thickness. I could not detect any connexion or adhesion between the kidney and its cyst; for the former could be drawn out, and removed without any resistance being experienced: but between it and the interior of the cyst was a thin stratum of purulent-looking fluid. This kidney was evidently smaller than the right one; its surface was soft and flocculent, and this looseness of strueture extended towards the centre of the organ, becoming, however, gradually less marked. On making a section of it, the tubular portion, in its interior, presented a natural firmness and structure; but it appeared redder than usual, as if it had been lately engorged.

Exp. 9. In a middle-sized strong animal, the right renal vein was exposed, and a ligature tied at such a distance from the vessel as not immediately to impede the flow of blood through the latter. The ureter was also tied. At the end of eighteen hours, the animal was killed. The urine found in the bladder was not albuminous; that in the right ureter seemed nearly pure blood. The left kidney weighed 64 grs.; the right, 182 grs.

Exp. 10. The left renal vein of a full-grown fat rabbit was, in the same manner, included within a loose loop, and the animal killed at the end of an hour. The bladder contained bloody urine. The right kidney weighed 90 grs.; the left, 170.

Exp. 11. The left renal vein being exposed, in a

small healthy rabbit, the artery was seen to pass obliquely behind it, rendering it very difficult to isolate the former vessel. A thread was passed around both, and tied so as to enclose both within a loose loop. Eight hours afterwards, the animal was alive and well. At the end of twenty-four hours, I found it dead and cold. The left kidney was much enlarged; it was enveloped in a distinct cyst, apparently formed of the surrounding cellular tissue, which had been infiltrated with blood and lymph. Except at one point, where the kidney had been slightly scratched, there was no adhesion between that organ and its investing membrane; in fact, they were separated from each other by a small quantity of serous fluid. After reflecting this tunic, an inner one (which I imagined to be the proper capsule) appeared, and, like the former, could be detached from the surface of the gland: thereby proving satisfactorily the real existence of a second membrane. The bladder contained about a drachm of clear urine, which was moderately but distinctly albuminous.

Exp. 12. A precisely similar operation was performed on a rabbit of the same size, the vein alone being included in the loop; it died at the end of two days and a half. The left kidney was surrounded by a cyst similar to that met with in the last experiment; it adhered slightly at one or two points to the capsule; the latter could be stripped off the kidney, and the separate existence of the two membranes thus manifested. The external surface of the gland presented three or four white spots, resembling those of incipient suppuration or softening. The urine in the bladder was of a faint reddish tinge, and was very highly albuminous.

Class II.

DESIGNED TO ILLUSTRATE THE PECULIARITIES OF ARTERIAL DETERMINATION.

A.—Removal of one kidney.

Four animals, of the same age and size, and in similar condition, were selected. The operation was performed at the same time on all of them, and the left kidney weighed at the time of its removal.

Exp. 1. The left kidney of a healthy young rabbit was removed, the vessels being previously tied; it died at the end of twenty-four hours, partly from the shock of the operation, and partly from peritonitis. The urine in the bladder was not albuminous. The left kidney, when removed, weighed 20 grs.; the right, 25 grs.

Exp. 2. A similar operation was performed. The animal appeared quite well at the end of the second day, when I poured some cold water over it, with the view of increasing the determination to the remaining kidney; it seemed unable to bear the shock, and died about the end of the third day. The urine contained no albumen; but on adding an additional quantity of nitric acid, there was a copious precipitation of crystals of nitrate of urea. The left kidney weighed 21 grs.; the right, 26 grs.

Exp. 3. At the same period, after the operation, this animal was treated in the same manner as the last; it lived twelve hours longer than it. There was no albumen in the urine; nor did any deposit of urea take place on adding an equal quantity of nitric acid. The left kidney weighed 20 grs.; the right, 33 grs.

Exp. 4. Nine days and a half after the removal of its left kidney, this animal appeared quite well; it was then killed. The bladder contained a small quantity of urine, which yielded a faint cloudiness when treated with nitric acid. The left kidney weighed 21 grs.; the right, 50 grs.

Exp. 5. The left kidney of a middle-sized strong rabbit was removed, and the animal killed at the end of nine days. The left kidney was unfortunately not weighed; the right was evidently much enlarged. The urine in the bladder was not albuminous.

B.—Ligature of the aorta, below the origin of the renal arteries.

Exp. 1. In a small weak rabbit, the abdominal aorta was tied, from an incision on the right side of the spine, which added to the difficulty, and, consequently, increased the shock of the operation. There was immediate and permanent paralysis of the hinder extremities. The animal died about ten hours after the operation. Both kidneys appeared disproportionately large; each weighed 36 grs., and the tubular portion of each was reddened. The urine was tested with nitric acid. In a small quantity, there was no appearance of albumen; in a larger, some permanent opacity was produced, not removable by a slight excess of the acid.

Exp. 2. The aorta was tied, from an incision on the left side of the spine, in a middle-sized animal, in poor condition. There was immediate paraplegia, as in the last instance. Some hæmorrhage from the smaller vessels occurred. It was killed at the end of forty minutes. Both kidneys were of a lighter, or more rosy tint than natural; the tubular portion of each was reddened. The left weighed 4 grs. more than the right; probably from the lower origin of the left renal artery in this instance. The urine in the bladder was not albuminous.

C.—Ligature of the aorta and removal of one kidney.

Exp. 1. The aorta of a middle-sized animal, in poor condition, being exposed by an incision in the left lumbar region, it was grasped by a spring forceps of moderate power. The obstruction to the flow of blood was complete, for the artery visibly enlarged above the point of compression. The animal was then liberated, and its hinder extremities were seen to be paralysed, the useless limbs trailing after the rest of the body. The blades of the forceps were then separated, and carefully withdrawn, and the animal almost instantly regained the power of moving its limbs. A thread was then passed beneath the aorta, and a knot tied at such a distance from the vessel as not to obstruct the flow of blood. The left kidney was now removed; it weighed 33 grs. On laying it open, the tubular portion was reddened, and on dissecting off the lining membrane of the pelvis, the primary arterial divisions beneath it were seen to be imbedded in a quantity of clear lymph. The paralysis of the hinder extremities *never* returned. Four hours after the operation, it was alive, and hopping about. At the end of eighteen hours I found it dead. The right kidney weighed 35 grs. No lymph could be seen beneath the lining membrane of the pelvis. The bladder was distended with urine, which was not albuminous. The ligature hung quite loosely on the aorta, but some bloody lymph had been effused around it.

Exp. 2. In an animal of similar size to the last, and, like it, in very poor condition, the aorta, being exposed, was compressed by the same forceps, and the animal then set free. There was perfect paraplegia. The forceps being separated and withdrawn, it continued to lie in the same position, having its hinder extremities extended and useless, for a few seconds, and then suddenly sprung up with a bound, having perfectly regained the power of moving them. The aorta was then tied tightly, when the paralysis immediately returned, and continued unchanged till death. The left kidney being now removed, weighed 32 grs.; on laying it open, the redness of the tubular portion, and the effusion of lymph beneath the membrane of the pelvis, existed as in the previous case. The animal was alive four hours afterwards, and was found dead about eighteen hours after the operation. The right kidney weighed 32 grs., and presented precisely the same appearances as the left. The bladder was full of urine, which contained no albumen.

Exp. 3. The left kidney of a very weak small animal was removed, and the aorta exposed. Some difficulty was experienced in passing a thread around the latter, in consequence of a great quantity of citron-coloured serous fluid accumulating in the wound; it did not flow from the peritoneal cavity, but was a mere oozing from, or through the vessels. The blood was very poor; its want of viscidity, as felt by the fingers, was very remarkable. The aorta was tied tightly, producing instantly the ordinary paralysis. The animal was killed at the end of five minutes; but, from the absence of any unnatural appearance in the right kidney, I did not deem it necessary to examine the urine.

Exp. 4. The aorta of a healthy young rabbit being tied, produced, instantly, permanent paraplegia. The left kidney was then removed, and weighed 30 grs. At the end of eighteen hours, the animal was still alive, but apparently at the point of death; it was then killed. The right kidney being examined, was reddened in every part of its substance, and presented on its surface some slight spots of ecchymosis, but it only weighed 30 grs. The bladder contained about a drachm and a half of muddy red urine, which held bloody coagula suspended in it.

On testing the liquid portion with nitric acid, albuminous flakes were produced.

Exp. 5. The aorta being exposed, in a young healthy rabbit, was included within a loose loop. The animal continued to run about without any appearance of paralysis. The left kidney was removed at the same time, and weighed 35 grs. Twenty-seven hours afterwards, the power of motion was still unimpaired. At the end of the second day it was found dead. The right kidney weighed 42 grs. On tracing the aorta, it was seen to be embedded in a quantity of lymph, that had been thrown out round the thread, but the canal of the vessel was still pervious. The loop had been applied about half an inch below the origin of the right renal artery, which seemed rather enlarged. The bladder contained nearly two drachms of urine, which was highly albuminous, forming instantly a large coagulum on the addition of nitric acid.

Exp. 6. The aorta of a full-grown strong rabbit was tied tightly, and the left kidney removed; but the ligature round the vessels of the latter having become somewhat loosened, some active arterial hæmorrhage took place. This kidney was of a lighter tint than usual, and weighed 82 grs. The ordinary paraplegia was present. Three hours and a half after the operation, the animal was in the same condition, and was then killed. The right kidney was enlarged and reddened; it weighed 112 grs. The bladder was nearly empty, only two or three drops of bloody urine escaping from it. On tracing down the ureter, its upper portion was dilated to the extent of more than an inch. A coagulum of blood plugged up the lower end of this portion, and on removing it by the division of the tube, a few drops of bloody urine escaped, then some clearer fluid, then a white fibrinous coagulum, and, above all, some twenty drops of clear urine. On allowing the latter to fall into a watch-glass, without any admixture of the bloody urine, and then adding nitric acid, it was found to be very highly albuminous, instantaneous coagulation being produced by this test.

Exp. 7. The left kidney of a middle-sized rabbit, in rather good condition, was removed, and found to weigh 54 grs. The aorta was then tied, without any accident occurring, and was followed by the usual paralysis. This animal seemed to recover from the shock of the operation more quickly than some former ones; it was killed at the end of two hours. The right kidney weighed 85 grs.; it contained six or seven ecchymoses of various extent, in different parts of its substance, but chiefly on the surface; its colour was much lighter than in those experiments in which the engorgement of the organ was produced by venous obstruction. The bladder contained about a drachm of urine, which was bloody and albuminous.

(These experiments have been repeated by Professor Frerichs in Germany, on different animals, with precisely similar results. He also examined the urine microscopically, and found it to exhibit the fibrinous casts of the tubuli uriniferi, and the copious epithelial cells so often noticed in Bright's disease of the kidney, thus furnishing additional evidence of the influence of renal congestion in producing many of the most characteristic phenomena of that disease. He states conclusively, "It is therefore no longer doubtful that the obstruction of the current of venous blood in the kidneys produces, as a consequence, the passage of albumen, fibrine, and, finally, also of blood itself, into the urinary passages." He also confirms my experiments as to the similar changes in the composition of the urine effected by an increased determination of blood to the renal artery:—"By tying the aorta, and at the same time destroying a kidney, a constant transmission of considerable quantities of albumen into the urine is produced." He concludes, by expressing an opinion that, "In the explanation of pathological phenomena, these facts ought to be taken into careful consideration."*)

* Frerichs "Die Bright'sche Nierenkrankheit," pp. 276–8. Brunswick, 1851.

ON THE

MECHANISM OF ABSORPTION.

Necessity for due Performance of Circulation. — Experiments of Physiologists. — Experiments of Natural Philosophers. — Application of these to the Phenomenon of Vascular Absorption. — Absorption proportioned to the Velocity of the Fluid moving in Vessels. — This Doctrine accounts for several Healthy and Morbid Processes in the Economy.

[From the LANCET and MEDICAL GAZETTE of May, 1843.]

IN a memoir which was read before the Royal Medico-Chirurgical Society in February last, I attempted to prove, by a series of experiments, that a partial or complete obstruction to the passage of the blood through the smaller vessels of the body will cause the escape of its albuminous portion through their coats. In the present communication I wish to direct attention to the influence which the opposite condition of the circulation exercises in promoting the absorption of any fluids that may be placed in contact with the external surface of the vessels, or only separated from them by one or more membranes.

If we examine the facts brought forward to illustrate the process of absorption, we shall find that the following is, perhaps, the only general conclusion that can be safely drawn from them, viz.: —

That no substance can exert any influence on the whole system unless the circulation of the blood, through the vessels of the part to which it may be applied, is performed with a certain degree of activity.

That the circulation of the blood must precede and accompany the act of general absorption is, among many other instances, proved by the following experiments: —

1. Magendie divided all the parts of the thigh of an animal but the femoral vessels, and then inserted poison under the integuments of the limb. While the vein was compressed no symptoms appeared, but they were immediately produced when the return of the blood was unimpeded.

2. Emmert tied the abdominal aorta, and introduced poison into a wound in the foot, but at the end of seventy hours no effects had appeared. The vessel being then liberated the poison (prussic acid) acted within half an hour. I have repeated the experiment with precisely similar results. The aorta being compressed, a few drops of a strong solution of hydrosulphate of ammonia were introduced beneath the integuments of the thigh. At the end of seven minutes no symptoms of poisoning had appeared, but on then releasing the vessel the operation of the poison was immediately evident, and the animal was dead in less than a minute. A number of similar facts might be adduced in support of this point, but it will be sufficient to refer for them to any modern work on physiology.

This principle being established, we may, in the next place, proceed to inquire how the action of the circulation, in favouring absorption, is to be explained.

According to the laws regulating the transmission of *stagnant* fluids through membranes, exosmosis and endosmosis should be continually occurring through the coats of the vessels of the living body; and there undoubtedly analogous processes do take place. But it appears to me highly important that we should ascertain how far those laws are modified *when one or both fluids are in a state of motion.* However, Magendie, and all succeeding physiologists who have adopted his opinion, suppose that the external fluid permeating the membranous coats makes its way to the internal surface of the blood-vessel, and is *then* swept on by the current of the blood.

According to this hypothesis the chief part of the process of absorption is made to reside in some peculiar power possessed by the membranous coats of the vessels,—the circulating fluid itself being quite a secondary agent, though, as above stated, its motion is necessary for the action of any poison on the system at large.

To prove the truth of his opinion, Magendie performed an experiment. He passed a stream of water through a portion of carotid artery and jugular vein, having previously applied strychnine to the exterior of the vessels. In a few minutes the water discharged had acquired the bitter taste of the poison.

Now this experiment, considered by itself, throws little light on the mechanism of absorption; it merely proves that while a stream traverses a membranous tube any soluble matters placed on the exterior of that tube will be absorbed; but as to the relative influence of the stream and the membrane in accomplishing that end, we are left altogether in the dark. He referred the whole of the transmitting power to the membrane, but the same experiment will, I think, prove equally well the influence of the stream in increasing that power.

It has long been known that a fluid, while traversing any porous vessel, will draw in a considerable quantity of air, which is liberated when the fluid is again at rest.

I now proceed to quote an experiment from Sir John Leslie's "Elements of Natural Philosophy," vol. i. p. 364:—

If a cylinder, "one inch in diameter, and three inches long, be fitted into an orifice at the bottom of a cistern, and on its upper side, at the distance of half an inch from its origin, a narrow arched glass tube inserted, the long end of which is carried down to a basin of water, three feet below the insertion of the other end,—when a stream traverses the cylinder with a velocity of nine feet per second, it will raise the water up the glass tube to the height of two feet, and if the tube be shortened within that limit, the basin will in a short time be emptied of the stagnant fluid." I have now several times repeated this experiment, and with a rapid stream the results were always in accordance with the above statement. Having filled a wine-glass with coloured fluid, and having connected its contents (by means of a bent tube twelve inches long) with the interior of a pipe half an inch in diameter, I found that the glass was drained of the stagnant fluid in less than two minutes after the stream was turned through the pipe.

I may refer to the same page for a proof of the statement that this imbibing power of the stream is proportioned to its velocity.

I will mention one other proof. While a cistern is full the rate of discharge and consequent velocity of the stream through the orifice at its bottom will, of course, be greatest. Now, if the apparatus above described be fitted into a pipe connected with this orifice, it will be found that the stagnant fluid will rapidly rise to a certain height in the glass tube; but as the depth of the column of water in the cistern diminishes, the fluid in the tube will oscillate and fall till the stream becomes so tardy as not to exert any marked influence on the stagnant fluid.

Having now proved the existence of this power, and also that it is proportioned to the velocity of the stream, the first step towards the application of this principle to the explanation of the process of absorption in the living body, is to show that the same force, whatever it may be, will act through one or more membranes.

Accordingly, the short end of the glass tube being covered with membrane and its long end immersed in a coloured fluid, I found that within five minutes after the stream had commenced to flow, the whole of the air present in the tube (which was twelve inches long and its bore one-fourteenth of an inch wide) had been absorbed and its place supplied by the coloured fluid. A continued slow ascent of the latter was still proceeding when I was compelled to stop the experiment. I afterwards repeated it, covering the short end of the tube with two membranes instead of one, but using a tube several inches shorter than in the last case, and found that there was a very slow, but steady and constant, flow of the fluid towards the stream; the fluid which thus traversed the tube being opposed in its flow by gravity, and being itself of greater specific gravity than that of the water constituting the stream.

By these direct experiments, and from a careful consideration of the chain of indirect evidence furnished by a number of morbid and healthy actions that are known to occur in the bodies of animals, I am, I think, justified, even in the present incipient stage of the inquiry, in making the following statement.

That as it has been shown that the effusion of albuminous matters through the coats of the vessels of the living body is produced by and modified in its nature according to the degree of the compression of the blood contained within them, this action being independent of and even in opposition to the ordinary laws of exosmosis as deduced from experiments on *stagnant* fluids; so I believe the chief part of the process of absorption in animals to arise from and depend on a force existing within the blood-vessels, that force being generated by, and proportioned to, the velocity of the moving mass by which, in a healthy state, they are incessantly traversed.

That something like a suction-power acts in promoting or causing absorption is undoubtedly a very old opinion, and the truth of this remark is evident in the literal signification of the very word. But so far as my present knowledge extends, all previous theories have referred that power either to the enlargement of the chest in inspiration or to the dilatation of the ventricles.

Now, while readily admitting the influence of these two actions in facilitating the return of venous blood, and thereby indirectly favouring absorption, I cannot think that they exercise any immediate effect in promoting the entrance of extraneous matters through the coats of the smaller vessels.

But if, on the other hand, we suppose this suction-power, whatever its precise nature may be, to be caused by and reside in the stream of blood, to be greatest wherever the current of the latter is most rapid, to be increased in its activity by whatever accelerates the velocity, and diminished by whatever induces a retardation, of the circulation through the part, then we shall have a principle of action, at once simple and efficacious, in perfect accord with the established laws of matter, and by the operation of which many morbid and healthy phenomena of the human body can be satisfactorily explained and readily understood.

In the present stage of the inquiry I shall not attempt to make many applications of this principle, but content myself with briefly alluding to some facts which seem to corroborate the doctrine herein sought to be established.

Magendie proved that a state of plethora retarded, and one of depletion promoted, absorption. These two conditions of the system are evidently attended by two opposite degrees of activity of the circulation. For when the mass of blood is much augmented, the obstacles which naturally oppose its free passage through the smaller vessels are materially increased, at the same time that the action of the heart is slower and more laboured than in health. Consequently, the proportion then existing between the moving power and the mass to be moved is unfavourable to a rapid circulation; and we may thus explain the slower action of poisons after he had injected a quantity of water into the veins. Whereas, after bleeding, or any other large evacuation, the whole of the arteries contract as the quantity of blood in the system diminishes, so as to form a series of narrower tubes, and the heart being relieved of a part of its load, after the first shock is over, increases the rapidity of its contractions so much that a more rapid circulation of the blood must necessarily result.

There are two parts of the animal economy where the process of absorption is actively carried on, and where some beautiful modifications of this principle are exemplified. I have said that compression of the blood within its vessels causes effusion; it should follow, therefore, that the compression of an external fluid against membranous tubes, while traversed by a rapid stream, will promote absorption; and such is known to be the case. The influence of pressure in causing the absorption of morbid effusions in the human body is well known, and its application is seen in daily practice. In the intestines, through which the bodies of animals obtain all their nourishment, some provision for increasing the absorbing power of the blood-vessels was required, and is accordingly there found. Their peristaltic action keeps up a steady continued pressure of the chyme against the vessels, thereby regulating, to a certain extent, the quantity of fluid effused from the latter, at the same time that their calibre is diminished and the velocity of the blood traversing them consequently increased. It has been an interesting problem in physiology to explain how the fœtus is nourished by the maternal blood without any direct vascular communication existing. On viewing the maternal vessels, it is evident, from their increased diameter, great length, and tortuous arrangement, that the circulation through them must be much retarded; while, on the other hand, the shorter circuit of the fœtal blood and the more rapid contractions of the fœtal heart, tend to prove that the velocity of the fœtal blood during its passage through the placental vessels is much greater than that of the maternal circulation in the same part.

Since, therefore, it has been shown that the absorbing power of a stream is proportioned to its velocity, it should follow that when two currents of blood moving with different degrees of velocity are in juxtaposition with each other, being separated merely by two thin membranes, the more rapid stream will not only draw in any fluid that may have been already effused by the other, but may even directly increase the rapidity of that exudation.

In whatever part of the body the course of the vessels is tortuous, or their coats are relaxed, a retardation of, and consequent obstruction to, the circulation of the blood results, effusion takes place, and absorption is performed very slowly if at all; and with opposite conditions of course we have opposite effects. We can thus understand why the surface of old ulcers should absorb more freely than that of recent ones; why a ligature tied round the limb impedes the action of poisons; and why the same beneficial result attends the application of a cupping-glass over a poisoned wound. In short, throughout the whole body the two antagonistic processes of effusion and absorption are constantly in operation, the preponderance of the one or the other in any particular part being regulated by the facilities or impediments afforded to the passage of the blood through the smaller vessels of that part. And I believe that absorption takes place chiefly in the smaller vessels, being facilitated there by the tenuity of their coats and the rapidity of the stream traversing them. As before stated, I consider these two processes to be in their nature and causes essentially different from those usually understood by the terms endosmosis and exosmosis, and to be in a great measure independent of the laws regulating the transmission of *stagnant and uncompressed fluids* through membranes.

ON CERTAIN POINTS IN THE

MECHANISM AND PHYSIOLOGY OF THE CIRCULATION OF THE BLOOD.

[From the LONDON MEDICAL GAZETTE, 1844.]

SINCE the discovery of the circulation by Harvey, numerous and important functions have at different periods been assigned to it; and every year tends to add to their number. Thus, among other uses, it is generally recognised as the instrument by which nutriment is conveyed to every part of the system, and effete and noxious matters are transmitted to their proper points of discharge. But while all agree in regarding the circulation as a chief means of intercommunication and transport, there is an extensive and highly important class of functions, in the production of which this agent is, by the majority of physiologists, considered to exert but a partial and secondary influence. The functions to which I allude, all involve either the discharge through the coats of the minute blood-vessels of certain matters previously present in the blood; or the entrance of various external substances into the mass of ciren-lating fluid. Under the former of these divisions may be mentioned—

1st.—Nutrition, or that process by which a constant supply of their proper aliment is furnished from the blood-vessels to the different tissues of the body.

2ndly.—Secretion and excretion: and in the performance of these functions we may presume that the mechanism of *effusion* is similar, whether the matters discharged by the secreting organs are separated directly from the blood, or are maturated in an intermediate series of cells.

3rdly.—Under the term vascular absorption, I would comprise all those functions which consist essentially in the entrance within the blood-vessels of various external substances.

Of the forces which produce this passage of fluids into and out of the blood-vessels, and of the laws by which these forces are regulated, we know very little with certainty. The explanation at present most generally received is that advanced by Magendie, Fodera, and other French physiologists, viz. that all these functions are referable to the power of capillarity inherent in the porous coats of the vessels, and are thus analogous to the phenomena of endosmosis and exosmosis.

To this doctrine it may be objected—

1st.—That the majority of experiments adduced in its support were performed with fluids stagnant, and subjected to equal pressure—conditions which can seldom or never occur, in precisely an equal degree, to the fluids situated on either surface of the minute blood-vessels of the living body.

2ndly.—This hypothesis does not explain how, in particular organs, one or other action is permitted wholly to preponderate; and it is quite certain that the two processes of imbibition and absorption do not proceed simultaneously, and with equal degrees of activity, in all the organs of the body, and in every part of the smaller sanguiferous tubes; for if an equal amount of interchange took place in the animal body wherever two fluids are separated from each other by a thin membranous septum, we should, in this case, continually incur the danger of being poisoned by the re-absorption of excreted noxious matters.

3rdly.—The same viscidity and cohesiveness, which impede so powerfully the passage of the blood through its smaller vessels, must oppose a still greater amount of resistance to that minute separation of its particles which is necessary for the effusion of albumen through the invisible pores of membrane. And the difficulty of applying this power to the explanation of certain of the functions in question is still further increased by the fact that, in experiments with viscid fluids, they are found to imbibe much more than they exhale.

It is true that the ordinary physical properties of membrane are said to be modified in the living body by peculiar physical causes, such as heat, electricity, &c. But from a consideration of these, and other reasons that might be mentioned, it would appear that this doctrine tends to invest the porosity of membrane, considered as a cause of motion, with much greater and more varied powers than it has been experimentally proved to possess; at the same time that the functions which are referred to those powers remain as unintelligible as ever. Nor can the mechanism of these processes be fully understood, till some force more active, more manageable, and more comprehensible than any yet advanced, is applied to the elucidation of the subject.

In the course of the following remarks I shall endeavour to demonstrate that such a force does exist in the circulation of the blood; and that this agent produces all the effects in question by directly or indirectly occasioning a disproportion between the amount of pressure acting on the internal and external surfaces of the minute blood-vessels. The researches on which this opinion is based were undertaken with no other object in view than the discovery of the laws by which the passage of substances into and out of the blood-vessels is regulated. I have at present therefore nothing to say concerning the means by which the different tissues and cells imbibe and assimilate their nutriment, nor of the mode in which the embryo obtains a supply of plastic matter previously to the existence of its circulation.

In these cases, the capillarity of the investing membranes may, perhaps, in the absence of any more active force, still be considered as the chief instrument employed for this purpose.

On examining the apparatus contrived for the passage of the blood to and from the heart, we observe considerable differences to prevail in the structure of the two great systems of blood-vessels, and in the course of the currents through them.

Thus, the large arteries are thick, strong, and highly elastic, while the coats of the veins are much thinner, their structure more porous, and their elasticity less marked.

Again, the arterial blood passes from one great trunk, through several intermediate branches, into an infinite number of minute twigs; whereas, in the veins, innumerable small currents meet in more capacious vessels, by the convergence of which two or three large streams are ultimately formed.

It may be further remarked, that the arterial blood encounters numerous obstacles to its free passage into the veins; whereas, in the latter vessels, as a general rule, every facility is afforded in order to secure the free return of the vital fluid. A consideration of these and other peculiarities, therefore, naturally suggests the opinion that the two great systems of blood-vessels are in health subservient to totally distinct, if not absolutely opposite, functions; and I shall now proceed to consider the facts which bear upon this conjecture.

Part I.

OF THE USES SERVED IN THE ANIMAL ECONOMY BY THE VARIOUS IMPEDIMENTS WHICH THE BLOOD ENCOUNTERS DURING ITS PASSAGE FROM THE VENTRICLES INTO THE VEINS.

The existence of numerous impediments to the free passage of the arterial blood is a fact so generally known and acknowledged, as to render unnecessary anything more than a brief mention of some of the most important obstructing causes.

The first to be considered is the arborescent arrangement of the arteries; which not only increases the surface of the vessels, and thus augments the friction, but also implies the division of the main current into as many minute streams as there are arterial twigs. The impediment arising from this cause must be materially augmented by the great viscidity of the blood; for the cohesion existing between its particles will oppose a considerable resistance to their necessary separation from each other.

2ndly.—We have the obstacles to the flow of blood occasioned by gravity—the weight of adjacent parts—the friction consequent on the angular origin and tortuous course of the arterial branches—muscular contraction—the resistance of the blood previously contained in the vessels, and some of minor importance.

3rdly.—The arterial blood, before entering the capillaries, has to encounter the impediment to its passage caused by the contractility of the smaller arteries and capillaries. In mentioning this vital property of the minute vessels as a chief obstacle to the progress of the arterial blood, I would beg to remark—1st, that our estimate of the aggregate amount of resistance opposed to the blood's passage through the small arteries is to be drawn from an examination of that encountered by the separate streams; and not from a vague calculation as to the relative areas of the aorta, and of its terminal branches; and 2ndly, that as the contractility of the small arteries and capillaries can, during its action, only cause a diminution in the area of the tubes which they form, and as that power of contraction is more marked in the distal part of the arterial twigs than at their point of origin from the main branch, it should follow that each minute stream of arterial blood will, if there be any difference in this respect, rather flow from the wider to the narrow portion of the tube.

Now the existence of these obstacles being undoubted, and their sum being so very considerable, are we to regard them as defects in the constitution of the circulation—unavoidable perhaps, but nevertheless involving a certain loss of power which might otherwise have been usefully employed in propelling the blood? And if the mere passage of that fluid through its vessels be deemed the sole intelligible part of the circulation, if we are to forbear from inquiring in what manner it produces its known beneficial effects upon the system, I do not see how some such supposition is to be avoided. But since it is possible that these very impediments to the circulation may in reality be contrivances adapted to the performance, by it, of some important functions, we are, I think, required, were it but in acknowledgment of the universal wisdom of nature's plans, to pause before we pronounce these apparent imperfections altogether inoperative, or disadvantageous. It therefore remains for us to inquire whether any peculiarity in the physical condition of the arterial blood is induced by the existence of these obstructing causes. And supposing this question to be answered in the affirmative, it will still remain to determine how far that physical condition of this portion of the vital fluid is subservient to any physiological uses.

The first effect resulting from the peculiar form, arrangement, and vital properties of the arteries, is a diminished rate of discharge of blood from the minute arterial ramifications into the capillaries and veins. And this is a necessary consequence of the established laws of hydraulics. For as any impediment to the passage of a fluid along its containing tube is known to diminish the rate of discharge from that tube, so, in like manner, must the impediments to the passage of blood through the small arteries cause the quantity of fluid leaving those vessels in a given time to be much less than what would escape from them in the same time, supposing those obstacles not to exist.

The only objection which strikes me as likely to be urged in opposition to this view is that embraced in the old opinion, that the arterial blood flows from the narrow to the wide portion of a conical tube, in consequence of the aggregate area of the minute arteries being greater than that of the aorta. But even if this statement were correct—though its truth has certainly not been satisfactorily demonstrated—it is nevertheless quite clear, that the obstacle to the blood's passage occasioned by the minute subdivision of the main current of viscid fluid, will more than counterbalance any advantage which might otherwise have been derived from the jointly increased calibre of the smaller arteries. So that the practical result, viz. the rate of discharge of blood from those vessels, will, as before stated, be precisely similar to what would be obtained were the arterial blood really to flow from the wide to the contracted portion of a tube.

The arrangement of the system of arterial tubes is therefore such as to present greater facilities for the entrance of blood, at one end, from the heart into the aorta, than for its discharge at the other, from the small arteries and capillaries into the veins.

And consequently, if the ventricle invariably expelled the whole of its contents at each contraction, there would, during an excited action of the heart, be so great a disproportion between the rates of influx and efflux of the arterial blood, as to render a rupture of some of the containing vessels almost inevitable. But it appears to me that this evil is *to a certain extent* guarded against by the following simple provision—viz. that the opposition to the entrance of fresh fluid from the left ventricle into the aorta increases in a direct ratio to the amount of disproportion between the rates of influx and efflux of the arterial blood. This opposition to the flow of blood from the heart arises from the backward pressure of the mass of aortic blood, which, after distending the arterial walls, is by their reaction driven back upon the aortic orifice of the ventricle. And as the extent to which the aortic walls are distended is, cæteris paribus, proportioned to the quantity of blood detained in it at the time, and as the quantity of this blood is again wholly dependent upon the preponderance of the influx over the efflux of arterial blood, so it follows that whatever increases the disproportion between the rates of influx and efflux of that blood will at the same time add to its backward pressure, and thus impede the flow of fresh blood from the ventricle.

The condition which, in a healthy state of the body, regulates the efflux of blood from the arterial system, is evidently the contractility of the small arteries and capillaries—a force influenced by the nervous system, and known to be of varying activity;—while the influx of blood is still more distinctly referrible to the contractions of the ventriele.

Now if this cavity of the heart invariably emptied itself at each stroke, we might readily estimate the rate of influx of the arterial blood by ascertaining the number of its pulsations; but, from the previous reasoning, it appears more probable that the ventricle does not always expel the whole of its contents at each contraction, and that the extent to which it does so, at any one time, mainly depends upon the relative quantity of blood then contained within the aorta. For when the quantity of this detained blood, and the consequent distension of the aorta, are very much diminished, as after loss of blood, then the opposition to the influx of fresh fluid from the ventricle is so much reduced, that it may readily empty its contents into the aorta; but if the heart's action be suddenly increased at a time when the quantity of blood detained in the aorta is already very considerable, each contraction will but add to the resistance opposing the entrance of fresh fluid into the arterial system, and will thus prevent the ventricle from expelling the whole of its contents at each pulsation.

As the causes impeding the flow of blood through the arteries exist throughout the whole extent of that system of tubes, increasing in their amount of opposition until it reaches a maximum in the minute vessels immediately continuous with the veins, it follows that the act of accumulation or detention of a quantity of blood behind each impeding surface will also continue in operation from the origin of the aorta to a point corresponding with the most contracted portion of the capillaries.

The blood thus detained in the arterial system, being prevented from moving readily forwards by the impediments so often referred to, while it at the same time receives an onward impulse from each successive wave of blood which leaves the ventricle, must necessarily exist in a state of compression, and will, consequently, exert a certain amount of outward or lateral pressure. If the obstruction to the blood's passage through the arteries were complete, then the accumulated fluid would of course be stagnant, and, like all other stagnant fluids, would transmit the whole of the impelling pressure equally in all directions. But as the obstacles occurring in the arteries present only a partial obstruction to the blood's passage through those vessels, the distending force of the arterial blood cannot be estimated till we have previously determined in what proportion the lateral pressure of a fluid is increased by the existence of any impediment to its free discharge from the containing tube. The following experiments, though rude and not sufficiently extended for the finer purposes of physics, may perhaps enable us to form some idea of the rate of increase in the lateral pressure of a fluid under these circumstances.

Exp. 1. I took a small wooden vessel, holding about three gallons of water, and fitted, horizontally, to its lower part, a cylindrical tin pipe, three inches long and half an inch in diameter (Fig. 1). On the

FIG. 1.

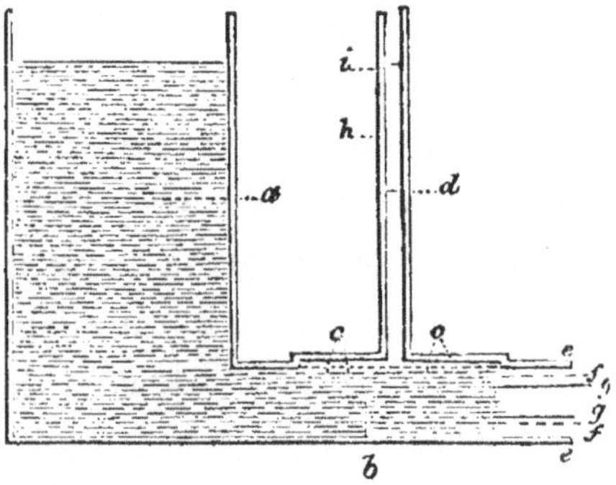

a, The reservoir.

b, The horizontal pipe communicating through the minute apertures, *c c*, with the interior of the vertical glass tube, *d*.

e e, The external orifice of the horizontal pipe, of its full diameter.

f f, The same reduced in diameter from $\frac{1}{2}$ to $\frac{1}{3}$ of an inch.

g g, The same still further reduced to $\frac{1}{6}$ of an inch.

h, The height to which the water rose in the glass tube when the diameter of the external orifice was reduced to *f f*.

i, Its height at the time that the external orifice was contracted to *g g*.

upper surface of this pipe, ten small holes, each about one twelfth of an inch in diameter, were made at an equal distance from each other, so as to extend along the whole length of the pipe, with the exception of half an inch at either end: over these apertures an arched piece of tin was soldered, from the centre of which projected upwards a short branch, and into it was fitted, vertically, a glass tube, twenty inches long and one quarter of an inch in diameter.

The junction of this tube with the short vertical branch was made water-tight, and the descent of the former into the main passage, through the tin pipe, was of course rendered impossible by the minuteness of the communicating apertures. The wooden vessel or reservoir was then filled with water to a height of twelve inches above the entrance of the tin pipe, and the column in it was maintained at the same elevation by the constant addition of fresh fluid. On removing a plug which had been previously placed at the inner orifice of the tin pipe, the water rushed through the latter, and escaped in a jet, sweeping, in this course, across the minute apertures which communicated with the interior of the glass tube.

During the whole of the time that this flow continned, there was no ascent of water in the glass tube; showing that, if the stream traversing the tin pipe did exert *any* lateral pressure, its amount was so inconsiderable as to be incapable of raising a column of water to the height of one inch; for it would then have been perceptible in the tube.

Exp. 2. The apparatus being in every other respect untouched, a short straight tube, one-third of an inch in diameter, was so fastened into the centre of the outer orifice of the tin pipe as entirely to prevent any escape of fluid from the latter, with the exception of that which passed through this smaller tube. The height of the column maintained in the reservoir was the same as in the last experiment, viz. twelve inches. On then allowing the water to enter the tin pipe, and escape freely through its narrowed extremity, it instantly rose in the vertical glass tube to a height of nine inches, and continued at that elevation as long as the same column of water was maintained in the reservoir. On allowing the latter to fall to ten inches, the same proportion was still observed between its height and that of the fluid in the glass tube, which had, during the same time, fallen to seven and a half inches.

Exp. 3. Every other condition being precisely similar, the tube one-third of an inch wide was withdrawn from the outer orifice of the tin pipe, and replaced by one one-sixth of an inch in diameter. On the re-admission of water into the tin pipe, it instantly rose in the glass tube to within half an inch of the height of the column in the reservoir, viz. to eleven and a half inches, though a jet one-sixth of an inch in diameter was, at the same time, escaping through the outer orifice of the horizontal pipe. A finger was now placed upon the inner orifice of this pipe, where it projected into the reservoir, and slowly drawn over it, so as gradually to diminish the area of the stream of water entering it; and it was observed that, in proportion as that diminution took place, there was a corresponding fall of the fluid in the glass tube, till, with a certain extent of closure of the inner orifice, there ceased to be any ascent of water in the vertical tube.

When the column in the reservoir was allowed to fall, the same proportion between its height and that of the water in the glass tube was still preserved, the difference never exceeding half an inch.

In these experiments it was very evident that the

amount of lateral pressure exerted by the water traversing the horizontal pipe, as measured by the height of the column in the glass tube, was altogether dependent on the degree of facility afforded to the passage of the fluid through that pipe, by the relative areas of its inner and outer orifices.

While the conditions affecting the influx and efflux were equal, the lateral pressure was very inconsiderable; but when the discharge was diminished by the application of an impediment to the outer orifice alone, then the lateral pressure increased in a very rapid ratio. Thus, in the second experiment, a diminution in the diameter of the outer orifice, from one-half to one-third of an inch, increased the lateral pressure of the contained fluid from something less than a column of water one inch in height to that of one nine inches high, which was equal to three-fourths of the whole impelling force; and in the last experiment, a diminution of the diameter of the external orifice to one-third, viz. from one-half to one-sixth of an inch, caused the lateral pressure of the fluid in the horizontal pipe to approach to within half an inch of that of the impelling column.

Before applying these principles to the fluid contained in the arteries, I may be allowed to repeat a former observation, viz. that whatever proportion the area of the aorta may bear to that of the sum of its terminal branches, the obstacles preventing the free passage of blood through the latter will diminish its rate of discharge from them as virtually as though their joint calibre were actually less than that of the main trunk; and as the amount of lateral pressure exerted by a moving fluid is wholly regulated by the relative facilities afforded to its passage into, and out of, the containing tube, so the various obstacles opposing the free course and discharge of the arterial blood will increase the lateral pressure of that fluid as effectually as the diminution of the external orifice of the pipe did in the foregoing experiments. The truth of this latter statement may also be proved by actual experiment.

Exp. 4. Thus, having connected with the same reservoir a leaden pipe, a yard long, perfectly straight, of uniform calibre, and maintained in the horizontal position, I bored a small hole on its upper surface, at the distance of a few inches from its commencement. A full stream being then allowed to flow through it, there was no escape of water from this aperture, showing that the lateral pressure exerted by the moving fluid was at a minimum. I now bent, laterally, the external half of the pipe, so as to cause it to describe a gradual curve, the horizontal position being apparently unaffected. But when the stream was again permitted to traverse it, the lateral pressure of the fluid detained behind the curve had increased so much as now to cause a small jet to escape through the aperture.

It is therefore evident that, in addition to contraction, any of those other peculiarities in the form and arrangement of tubes, which are known to diminish their power of discharge, will also increase the lateral pressure of the fluid contained behind the impeding portions of the tube; and as it has, moreover, been shown that the amount of lateral pressure increases in a very rapid ratio on the application of any impediment to the free discharge of fluid from a tube, so it is rendered probable that the outward or distending pressure of the arterial blood is very considerable.

A question here arises as to the proportion which this lateral pressure of the arterial blood bears to the impelling power of the heart. The data which we possess may perhaps be deemed insufficient to warrant a positive answer, but, for the following reasons, I should imagine that these forces must generally be very nearly equal. The onward impulse of the arterial blood is supposed, from experiments performed on animals with the hæmadynamometer, to be equal, in man, to a column of the same fluid eight feet high. Poiseuille has, moreover, found this impulse to be nearly equal in the chief arterial branches. Now it follows, from the arborescent arrangement of this system of tubes, that the force of the blood entering the carotid artery must be nearly the measure of the lateral pressure of the aortic blood; and as the impulse of the blood entering the femoral artery, which, in direction, is continuous with the aorta, is no greater than that of the blood driven into the carotid, which is a lateral branch, it would appear that the mass of aortic blood presses equally in all directions, its lateral being equal to its onward pressure.* And, from the facts and arguments

* An experiment with the hæmadynamometer, on the renal artery, which arises from the aorta at a right angle, would remove all doubt on this point.

before mentioned, it is equally evident that this great lateral pressure of the fluid contained in the arteries can only be occasioned by the existence of a considerable difference between the relative facilities afforded for the influx and efflux of the arterial blood. As to the absolute force of the outward pressure, it must necessarily be subject to a still more extensive range of variation than that of the onward impulse derived from the heart's action; for it is equally affected by a change in the condition of the heart, or of the smaller vessels, both which changes are continually occurring. It may therefore, in the same individual, be at one time so slight as to be incapable of accomplishing its healthy uses, while, at another period, its distending power may be so considerable as to rupture some of the containing vessels, and thus threaten the destruction of life.

Having, I trust, satisfactorily proved that the whole mass of arterial blood exerts, during health, a considerable amount of outward or distending pressure, it now only remains for me to consider the second point which I proposed for examination, viz. whether any uses are served in the animal economy by the existence of this peculiar physical condition of the arterial blood; and in studying the physiological effects resulting from the operation of this force, it will be necessary to view it as existing, first, in the large arteries, and, secondly, in the minute arterial ramifications; for as the physical and vital properties of these vessels are essentially different, so will the application of the same distending force produce, in each, totally distinct phenomena.

The coats of the large arteries being dense, thick, and highly distensible, it is evident that an accumulation of blood in, and a forcible distension of, those elastic tubes, are the only effects which *can* occur from the detention within them of a quantity of highly compressed blood; for the escape of any portion of the contained fluid through the pores of the investing tissues is prevented by the great thickness and dense structure of the arterial tunics. It is also quite clear that any considerable accumulation of fluid can only take place in a tube when the walls of that tube are either flaccid or elastic; and that, in the latter case, the amount of the accumulation will, to a certain extent, be regulated by the distending power of the contained fluid. Since, therefore, various functions have been traced to the reaction of the elastic coats of the large arteries upon the distending force of the blood accumulated within them, and since that distending force has been shown to be no other than the lateral pressure of the arterial blood, we are, I conceive, now authorised to advance a step further, and say, that the functions in question are referrible to that lateral pressure as to the cause essentially producing them. The uses to which I more particularly allude are the equal distribution of the heart's impulse throughout the system, and the uniform and equable flow of blood through the capillaries and veins.

The properties of the smaller arteries are so very different from those of the vessels we have just been considering, that it is impossible to arrive at any satisfactory conclusion as to the effects induced in the former by the lateral pressure of the arterial blood, without determining and bearing in mind their distinctive peculiarities. They form a series of minute porous tubes, the coats of which, being highly contractile, are, in their healthy state, continually resisting the dilating pressure of the contained blood. In their relation, therefore, to that contained fluid, they represent so many rigid tubes. In them there is consequently no considerable accumulation of blood, nor do we find any functions performed by the elasticity of their investing tissues. But other and still more important effects are here induced by the lateral pressure of the arterial blood; for by the operation of this force there is a constant exudation of certain portions of the blood through the thin and porous coats of these minute vessels. For proofs, that compression of the blood in its smaller vessels will cause its effusion through the coats of the latter, and that the nature of this effusion is mainly regulated by the degree of that compression, I beg to refer to a paper contained in the last volume of the "Medico-Chirurgical Transactions:" in it will be found an account of some experiments in which, on directing an increased flow of blood through one renal artery (by obstructing the abdominal aorta and the blood-vessels of the other kidney), various component parts of the blood, viz. liquid albumen, fibrinous and coloured coagula, were found in the secretion of the organ thus inordinately supplied.

But the observation which bears most directly on the present point is this—that on examining these hypertrophied kidneys at the end of a few hours, I generally found the primary divisions of the renal artery imbedded in a quantity of liquor sanguinis, which the unnatural compression of the contained blood had expelled through their porous coats. Since, therefore, an additional degree of compression of the blood is capable of forcing its most viscid parts through the coats of vessels which, from their thickness, must oppose a very great resistance to the passage of fluid through their pores, we cannot, I think, avoid the conclusion, that a constant, though slow, and, to the naked eye, imperceptible, process of albuminous effusion through the thin porous coats of the minute arteries, is a necessary consequence of the existence in each of them of a distending column of blood. This process of effusion must necessarily take place whenever the pressure acting on the internal surface of the membranous tube is greater than that of the medium in which the tube or vessel is placed. And if, at any one point, the resistance of the medium be less than the outward or lateral pressure of the contained fluid, then effusion will occur at that point only. For so long as an amount of pressure greater than the dilating or lateral force of the contained fluid is applied on the external surface of a porous tube, the escape of that fluid through these minute lateral openings is evidently rendered as impossible as though the latter did not exist at all. In the living body the different tissues situated between the smaller blood-vessels, will represent the medium in which the latter are placed; and its resistance is evidently insufficient wholly to repress, though it probably limits within certain bounds, the tendency to effusion resulting from the compression of the blood in the smaller arteries. There is, therefore, from this source, a constant effusion of albuminous fluid into the intervascular spaces, and a supply of their proper nutriment is thus brought in immediate contact with the tissues of the body.

The absolute force of the lateral pressure of the blood contained in the smaller arteries of a particular part, will, equally with that of its onward pressure, be affected by any change in the area of the main arterial branch supplying them. Whatever, then, increases the supply of blood to a part, will, at the same time, increase the amount of lateral pressure acting on the inner surface of the coats of the small arteries of that part. The functions to which that lateral pressure is there subservient, must consequently, at this time also, be performed with unusual activity. And this reasoning is fully corroborated by the connexion invariably observed in health and in disease between the activity of the nutritive process and the rate of supply of blood to a part, as estimated by the number and calibre of the arterial trunks connected with it.

A similar preponderance of the pressure acting on the internal surface of the coats of the smaller arteries will undoubtedly assist in causing that separation or exudation of certain portions of the blood which constitutes the first stage in the processes of secretion and excretion. But as the capillaries, or intermediate vessels, are generally considered to exercise a still more important influence in the performance of these functions, it becomes necessary to consider how far the preceding views are applicable to this part of the circulating system. And on considering the endless varieties that are observed to prevail in different organs of the body, in respect to the relative length, number, arrangement, and connexion of these vessels with the adjacent arteries and veins, the following are those conclusions which appear to derive the greatest amount of support from the knowledge already possessed on the subject. Wherever, in an arborescent arrangement of vessels, the blood flows from a main branch into numerous collateral twigs, it must encounter more or less obstruction during its passage through the latter, and will consequently continue to exert a certain amount of lateral pressure until it has traversed the most contracted portion of the tubes. In those organs where a peculiar disposition of the vessels impedes the flow of blood from the capillaries into the veins, the same effect, viz. an increase in the lateral pressure of the capillary streams, must follow the diminished rate of discharge from the capillaries thus induced. The causes of this partial obstruction may be seated either in the capillaries themselves, or in the adjacent veins. In some organs, as in the Malpighian tufts of the kidney, their own arrangement is a considerable source of obstruction to the blood traversing the former vessels. And in other parts, a tortuous course of the neighbouring veins, gravity, or any other cause which impedes the return of venous blood, must, at the same time, induce a corresponding increase in the amount of lateral pressure of the blood contained in the capillaries supplying those veins. But it is chiefly in secreting structures that a disposition of parts so unfavourable to the free circulation of the blood through the capillaries is observed to occur. And on applying to these cases the law frequently referred to, viz. that any impediment to the passage of a fluid increases the amount of its lateral pressure, how are we to avoid the conclusion that this peculiar physical condition of the blood contained in the capillaries of secreting organs is a provision of nature for the accomplishment of the necessary exudation of certain portions of that compressed fluid? The blood contained in the capillaries of different parts of the body must therefore exert different degrees of lateral pressure according as the impediments to its passage into the veins are more or less considerable. An opinion formerly prevailed, supported by Keil, Hales, and other physiologists, that the extraordinary impediments to the free return of the venous blood, which are almost invariably observed in organs whose natural secretion is highly albuminous, are, in some way or other, connected with that peculiarity in the secreted fluid. Our knowledge of the minute anatomy of some of these organs is perhaps too imperfect to justify a positive conclusion on the subject. But the relative viscidity of an effused fluid being, by the facts before referred to, shown to depend upon the degree of compression endured by the blood contained in the small vessels; and the anatomical arrangement of the blood-vessels of these glands furnishing the impediment necessary for the compression of the blood circulating through them; these two considerations do appear to me sufficient to invest the old doctrine with a certain degree of probability. Physiologists are too unsettled in their views of the process of secretion to render necessary many additional remarks in applying the general law of effusion to this particular function. For whether the secreted matters be derived directly from the blood by a process of filtration, or are the results of various chemical changes effected in that effused fluid by the peculiar physical conditions to which it is subjected previous to its final discharge, or are generated according to vital laws in cells developed by vital powers similar to those concerned in the process of growth, or, as is perhaps most probable, by the conjoint operation of all these agencies, it is in each case equally evident that a constant supply of material will be required; and this supply can only be obtained from the blood-vessels of the secreting structure. It is unnecessary to recapitulate any of the former arguments for the purpose of proving that this effusion is due to the expelling force constituted by the lateral pressure of the blood contained in these vessels. But in closing this part of my subject, I may remark—1st, That the free surface on which secretion invariably occurs is another provision for facilitating the process of effusion, by substituting a less resisting for a denser medium: so that the vessels are less firmly supported on that side than on the rest of their circumference. The influence of a free surface, or of a loose structure, in facilitating effusion, is also strikingly exemplified in many of the phenomena of disease, and is clearly referrible to the diminished pressure then acting on the exterior of the minute blood-vessels: and, 2ndly, that the different degrees of compression which the blood endures in the capillaries of different glands will probably exercise considerable influence in modifying the nature of their secretion.

The capillaries distributed throughout the rest of the body will, at their junction with the minute arteries, assist the latter in the performance of the function of nutrition. The extent to which their share is limited, must, in each organ or structure, be mainly regulated by the relative facilities afforded to the passage of the blood into and from them. But in the following division of this memoir I shall mention some reasons in support of the opinion, that these vessels, more especially their terminating portions, are intimately connected with the adjacent venous radicles in the performance of the opposite function of absorption.

It may by some be considered that the foregoing views have too great a tendency to withdraw the functions of secretion and nutrition from the sphere of influence of the nervous system. But as it is generally acknowledged that the nerves possess the power of affecting the contractility of the blood-vessels so as to increase or diminish their calibre, and also that of the pores existing in their walls;

and as that increase or diminution in the relative size of different portions of the blood-vessels of an organ must necessarily be followed by corresponding changes in the amount of lateral pressure acting on the internal surface of those vessels: this doctrine is in reality calculated to establish a still more intimate connexion between the nervous system and these functions, by showing how the former is enabled to control the activity, and, at the same time, to modify to a certain extent the character, of the latter. I have now successively endeavoured to prove—

1. That the obstacles to the free passage of the arterial blood prevent the small arteries from discharging into the veins more than a limited quantity of blood in a given time.

2. That as the blood encounters fewer impediments in flowing into, than in escaping from, the arterial system, its rate of influx has a constant tendency to preponderate over its rate of efflux into the veins.

3. That the amount of this disproportion is ever varying; and that the evils which a great excess would occasion are probably in some measure obviated by the circumstance of the opposition to the influx of blood into the arterial system increasing in a direct ratio to the amount of disproportion between it and the rate of the efflux of blood into the veins.

4. That the whole mass of blood contained in the arterial system, from the heart to the most contracted portion of the capillaries, exerts a lateral pressure, the degree of which is altogether dependent upon

the relative facilities afforded to the entrance of blood into, and its discharge from, that system of vessels.

5. That the lateral pressure of the blood contained within the arteries is probably equal to its onward pressure, so that the arterial blood will press equally in all directions.

6. That this lateral pressure of the arterial blood is the force which maintains the large arteries in a state of distension, and thus enables their elastic walls so to re-act upon their contents as to be the means of accomplishing various useful purposes in the animal economy.

7. That the same force acting on the interior of the minute porous arteries causes that slight but constant exudation of certain portions of the blood which is indispensable to the performance of the important functions of secretion and nutrition.

8. That the blood contained in the commencement of the capillaries being subservient to the same uses, is also made to exercise some lateral pressure, the degree of which varies in different structures, but is probably never quite equal to that of the onward impulse of the same column of blood.

In conclusion, it may be remarked that as those impediments which limit the rate of the discharge of blood from the arterial system constitute the first and essential cause of all the subsequent phenomena, so the uses served in the body by the existence of these peculiar physical effects are, with them, clearly referrible to the same apparent imperfection in the mechanism of the circulation.

PART II.

OF THE MECHANISM OF ABSORPTION; IN WHICH IT IS ATTEMPTED TO TRACE THAT ACTION TO THE PECULIAR PHYSICAL CONDITIONS REGULATING THE PASSAGE OF THE BLOOD INTO AND THROUGH THE VEINS.

BEFORE mentioning the facts which appear to me calculated to illustrate the mechanism of the opposite function of absorption, it may be well briefly to review one or two of those opinions on the subject which have already been presented to the public.

I have previously had occasion to notice Magendie's general doctrine as to the transmitting power possessed by membranes; and have given some reasons for my disbelief in the sufficiency of that explanation of the various processes of exudation and absorption. The latter function, however, is by the same authority still more explicitly declared to depend upon an affinity of the vascular walls for the substances absorbed.* But while acknowledging the great value of many of the laws regulating animal absorption which have been established by the labours of this eminent physiologist, I cannot perceive that the experiments adduced in support of this particular doctrine do more than prove the porosity of membrane; for they appear mainly intended to show that the same interchange of fluids which takes place through inorganic porous septa, will, under similar circumstances, also occur through animal membrane.

* "Journal de Physiologic," t. i. p. 6.

And as this power was by Magendie himself considered as but *one* of the probable causes of vascular absorption*, it still remains to discover what other physical conditions assist in the performance of this function.

There is another view of absorption, which as it, in name at least, bears some resemblance to that which I shall presently advance, requires a moment's examination. I allude to the opinion of the late Sir D. Barry. The experiments of this gentleman prove very satisfactorily, that during each act of inspiration there is a rush of venous blood into the imperfect vacuum then formed within the thoracic cavity. On introducing a long glass tube into the interior of certain large veins, he also found that a coloured liquid, into which the lower end of the glass tube dipped, ascended in the latter to the height of several inches during each inspiration, and fell during the opposite act of expiration.

This ascent of the coloured fluid he conceived to be an act of absorption rendered visible by the glass tube, the lower end of which represented the open mouths of the absorbing vessels.† In observing that the sanguiferous and lymphatic vessels have a similar communication between their extremities and the thorax, he has apparently left out of considera-

* "L'affinité des parois vasculaires pour les matières absorbées étant supposée la cause, ou, si l'on veut, l'une des causes, de l'absorption," &c.—*Journal de Physiologie*, t. i. p. 8.

† "Experimental Researches on the Influence of Atmospheric Pressure upon the Blood in the Veins, upon Absorption," &c. By David Barry, M.D. &c. London, 1826

tion the yielding walls of the small blood-vessels, and the minuteness of the pores through which absorption occurs. This view of the process of absorption is moreover sufficiently refuted by one of the author's experiments. Thus he remarks that if the communicating tube be introduced into the femoral vein of a dog- or horse, and pushed no further, then the inspiration will produce no effect on the fluid in the cup; *because the relative vacuum in the thorax can be filled from the veins nearer to the chest.** This latter remark, and the admission that the operation of this partial vacuum within the thorax does not extend so far as the femoral veins, appear to be quite fatal to this view of absorption. And even if it could be shown that the expansion of the thorax exerts a *direct* influence on the passage of blood through the smaller veins, the immense disproportion existing between the area of the latter and that of the minute absorbing pores situated in their walls, would necessarily cause that influence to be exercised chiefly on the fluid contained within the larger tubes. His other experiments, in which the application of cupping-glasses over poisoned wounds prevented the action of the poison, cannot, in their physiological bearings, be considered as proving more than that an obstruction to the circulation through a part prevents absorption—a principle which has also been fully established by many other observers. It is now some time since the idea first occurred to me, that the same power of raising from a lower level, and drawing with it an external stagnant fluid,

* Op. cit., p. 15.

which Venturi found to be possessed by a rapid stream of water, might possibly also be in some measure exercised by the innumerable streams of blood which incessantly traverse the different structures of the animal body. If any analogous force did reside in the latter, then the total absorbing power thus obtained, must, from the number and rapidity of those currents, as seen under the microscope, be very considerable; and this force had certainly not yet entered into the consideration of physiologists. I repeated, with success, Venturi's chief experiment, viz. that of causing the ascent of a stagnant liquid in the long arm of a syphon, the short arm of which communicated with the interior of a pipe traversed by a rapid stream. And I also found the same ascent to occur, though much more slowly, when a membrane was tied over the orifice of the short arm, so that all communication between the interior of the syphon and the stream could only take place through the minute pores of the intervening membrane.

I had proceeded thus far in the inquiry, when circumstances prevented me from pursuing it further at that moment; but in May last, an abstract of my views on this subject, and of the grounds on which they rested, appeared in the "Medical Gazette."

Having since then performed a great number of experiments on various points connected with this process, I shall now proceed—

1st. to give a detailed account of some experiments, in which the substitution of yielding and compressible for rigid tubes (by assimilating the conditions of the observations to those known to exist in the living body) removes the chief, and, in my opinion, the only valid objection to this explanation of the function in question;

And conclude this part of my communication by endeavouring to elucidate the physical principles on which the action of absorption depends.

Exp. 1. A piece of the descending aorta of a horse, which formed a flexible yielding pipe, nearly cylindrical in shape, four inches long and one inch in diameter, was fastened horizontally to the lateral opening of the reservoir. Having previously closed all its collateral branches, with the exception of one, I fitted into the latter the short arm of an arched glass tube, the long arm of which dipped into a vessel containing coloured liquid. The internal orifice of the pipe was somewhat contracted in fastening it to the opening in the reservoir, so that its calibre at this point would be less than that of the rest of the pipe. During the passage of the stream through the latter, the coloured liquid rose in the glass tube, and on increasing the height of the impelling column the vessel containing the coloured liquid was speedily emptied. The outer orifice of the glass tube being then allowed to communicate freely with the external air, the jet issuing from the pipe instantly assumed the pulsating character; at the same time that the entrance of air into its interior caused a gurgling sound.

It now only remained to be shown that a stream traversing a flaccid membranous tube possesses the same power of absorbing an external stagnant fluid. But the difficulties preventing the successful performance of this experiment were much more considerable than any yet encountered; for the mere weight of the incumbent flaccid walls opposed so much resistance to the passage of fluid through the tube, that a copious exudation occurred through any lateral openings existing in it; and I could only obtain a satisfactory result by carefully observing, and in the performance of the experiment strictly adhering to, the conditions under which the return of venous blood is effected in animals.

The most important of these conditions may be thus stated:—

1. The different converging streams always flow from narrow into wider tubes.

2. Those flaccid porous tubes are placed in a dense medium, the pressure of which on their external surface is much greater than that of the atmosphere; for, in addition to this latter force, we have, in the living body, various other powers, the operation of which greatly increases the pressure acting on the exterior of the blood-vessels; as, for instance, the elasticity and contractility of the skin, the weight and lateral pressure of adjacent parts, muscular action, &c.

3. The walls of the terminating portion of the large venous trunks are strengthened and rendered comparatively rigid by their adhesion to the diaphragm, pericardium, and pleuræ.

4. The flow of venous blood into its proper receptacle—the right auricle—is facilitated by the

diminished pressure existing within the thorax during the act of inspiration.

It would be tedious to enumerate the different failures which I experienced in constructing an apparatus in which all these conditions should be observed. The following arrangement is that which proved most effectual; and the conditions under which the absorbing stream here acted appear to correspond very closely to those affecting the minute currents contained within the veins.

Exp. 2. The œsophagus of an ox, which formed a convenient membranous reservoir, was suspended vertically, and to its lower extremity was fastened a glass tube, fifteen inches long and one-fourth of an inch in diameter, the lower end of which was recurved, so that its orifice also looked directly upwards. The extent of tube involved in this curve was not above three inches, the length of the ascending portion being one inch. To the orifice of the latter was then fastened a piece of the small intestine of a fowl, which formed a membranous tube two inches long and about one-third of an inch in diameter; the other end of this flaccid tube was then attached to the short arm of a glass syphon one-third of an inch in diameter, the arms of which were respectively an inch and a half, and two inches and a half, long (Fig. 2).

The lower part of the descending, and the whole of the curved, portion of the first glass tube, the entire extent of the membranous tube, and the short arm of the syphon, were then placed in a glass vessel six inches deep, on the rim of which the angle of the syphon rested, so that the orifice of the long arm would discharge its contents on the exterior of the vessel (vide Fig. 2).

I must not omit to mention that the lower half of the membranous tube had been previously punctured

FIG. 2.

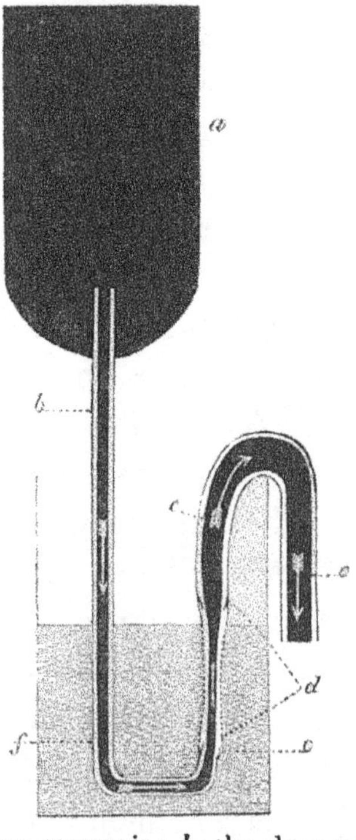

a, The membranous reservoir; *b*, the descending portion of the first glass tube; *c*, its ascending portion; *d d*, the membranous tube; *e e*, the glass syphon; *f*, the vessel containing the external coloured liquid.

with a fine needle, so as to make in it a great number of small lateral openings. This was done with the view of rendering the progress of the experiment more perceptible; for the great length of time required for the passage of an appreciable quantity of fluid through the minute pores of several layers of membrane would otherwise have added materially to the tedious character of the observation. It may also be observed, that this enlargement of the pores facilitated exudation quite as much as absorption; and in the living body the passage of fluids through the coats of the small blood-vessels is greatly promoted by their extreme tenuity, by the high temperature, and possibly by other favourable conditions.

The apparatus being thus arranged, a measured quantity of liquid was poured into the glass vessel, so as to reach nearly to the commencement of the short arm of the syphon, and a column of water, varying from three to five inches in height, was maintained in the membranous reservoir. It will be seen by a glance at the accompanying diagram that the fluid, after entering the first glass tube, and ascending from its curved portion, would then pass through the membranous tube, and reaching the short arm of the syphon, be finally discharged on the exterior of the vessel containing the stagnant fluid.

During its passage through the membranous tube, the stream was, by means of the lateral openings existing in the latter, enabled to communicate with the external stagnant liquid.

The calibre of the arched portion of the first glass tube had been considerably diminished by the flattening of the tube during the process of bending it; so that the stream escaping from it into the membranous tube was necessarily much less than one-fourth of an inch in diameter. But even this disproportion between the area of the stream entering the membranous tube, and that of the latter, did not prevent a rapid exudation from occurring whenever the height of the column in the reservoir exceeded two or three inches; and the following was the only method which I found effectual in obtaining constant absorption, viz. to grasp the upper end of the first glass tube, where it projected into the membranous reservoir, so as gradually to diminish its area until the stream escaping at the other end of the apparatus became reduced in size to a mere thread. And so long as the area of the stream entering the first glass tube was in this manner limited and regulated according to the height of the impelling column, absorption of the external stagnant fluid surrounding the membranous tube proceeded with tolerable rapidity. Thus in one experiment the quantity of stagnant fluid was in less than ten minutes diminished by three ounces; in another trial, its original quantity of nine fluid ounces was, during the passage of little more than half a pint of water through the apparatus, reduced to $4\frac{1}{2}$ ounces, or one-half. The stagnant fluid was occasionally coloured, and could then be seen to escape with the stream issuing from the syphon. At the commencement of the experiment there was invariably some effusion, until the long arm of the syphon became filled, when the process of absorption began, and, if uninterrupted, would gradually reduce the height of the stagnant fluid from the level of the short arm of the syphon to the junction of the membranous tube with the termination of the first glass tube. When a considerable extent of the membranous tube became in this manner exposed, globules of air also passed through its lateral openings, and escaped with the stream. While absorption was proceeding the membranous tube always became flattened, whereas during the occurrence of effusion it appeared distended, and more cylindrical in shape. In this apparatus the absorbing stream flowed almost directly upwards. In other cases, where the membranous tube was placed horizontally in a long shallow vessel, absorption of the external fluid occurred with the same rapidity so long as the same conditions were observed.

Having, by these experiments, proved that a stream, in passing through a flaccid membranous tube, can exercise an absorbing power, it now remains for me to show that in this rude apparatus there are represented the most important of those conditions which are known to affect the currents of venous blood. And these conditions may be considered in the same order in which they were before mentioned.

1. It is essential to the success of the experiment that the absorbing stream should flow from a narrow to a much wider tube. In this respect there is a marked analogy between the contrivance which repeated failure in these experiments suggested, and that arrangement of the minute veins and the contiguous portion of the capillaries by which the streams of blood traversing this part of the circulating system are made to operate in a precisely similar manner. For at this point innumerable small rapid streams are, throughout the body, per-

petually flowing from the capillaries into the contiguous venous radicles, the calibre of which is much greater than that of the vessels supplying them. At this point, therefore, the conditions are evidently favourable to absorption. And on tracing the course of the veins to their final termination in two or three large trunks, the individual streams are, in the same manner, constantly found to pass from narrow to wider tubes. In the smaller vessels this arrangement is obviously calculated to add to the absorbing power of the contained streams. In the large veins, the walls of which are too thick to be readily permeated by liquids, its chief use is apparently that of economising the impelling force of the vis à tergo, by diminishing friction.

2. The next point to be noticed is the medium in which the membranous tube was placed: and the necessity of a denser medium than atmospheric air was proved by a repeated observation of the fact, that when the membranous tube was unsupported, the whole of the fluid constituting the stream escaped through the lateral openings of the same apparatus which, when immersed in water, not only permitted the stream to traverse it freely, but also enabled the current to carry with it a considerable quantity of the external stagnant fluid. It is difficult to form any estimate of the average amount of pressure acting on the exterior of the blood-vessels of the living body. It must necessarily vary much in different animals, and in different parts of the same body. I have, however, been careful not to employ a greater amount of external pressure in these experiments than might reasonably be supposed to

exist in living animals. For in these experiments the force acting on the exterior of the membranous tube never exceeded the weight of a column of water six inches high, while in some cases the height of the external column was only one inch.

3. In imitation of the rigidity of the terminating portion of the large veins, the upper end of the membranous tube was fastened to a short arm of a bent glass tube. But this sudden transition from a flaccid to a perfectly rigid tube occasioned an inconvenience which will, to a certain extent, be avoided in the animal body, in consequence of the change being more gradual.

4. To compensate for the difficulties which a stream encounters in flowing against gravity, it became necessary to use the slight derivative power of a short syphon, and without this contrivance no absorption could be obtained with an ascending stream. As before mentioned, it has been shown by the experiments of Hales, and more recently by those of Sir D. Barry, that a similar derivative power acts during the expansion of the thorax. This force has been found capable of raising a column of water in a small glass tube to the height of twenty inches.

It might, from this latter circumstance, be imagined that the use of a more powerful syphon in the apparatus would have the effect of increasing the activity of the absorbing process. But I have satisfied myself, by repeated trials, that any material deviation from the above-stated proportions, whether increasing or diminishing the power of the syphon, rather impeded than promoted absorption. For when the derivative power was much increased, the gravitating column of water in the long arm diminished the pressure within the short arm so much, that the contiguous portion of the membranous tube was then forced against the orifice of the latter, so as entirely to close it. And this obstruction to the passage of the stream necessarily caused effusion through the lateral apertures of the membrane.

This inconvenience attending the employment of a more powerful syphon, would, I conceive, be experienced in a minor degree were the change from a flaccid to a rigid tube more gradually effected, as it is in the animal body. And to test the accuracy of this supposition, I repeated some of the former experiments with a more powerful syphon, having previously fastened to its short arm a piece of caoutchouc tubing half an inch long, and over that a membranous tube six inches in length. Although every other condition was the same as before, this slight alteration of the apparatus, by which the stream was made to pass from the membranous into the caoutchouc tube, and then into the glass syphon, facilitated the action of the latter so much, that a very rapid absorption of the external fluid occurred, though the lateral apertures in the membranous tube did not approach within three inches of the termination of the caoutchouc tube.

In explanation of this point, it may also be remarked, that though the derivative power exercised by the act of inspiration arises from the same immediate cause as that by which a syphon acts, viz. diminished pressure within the several recipient cavities, the mode of action of that cause nevertheless differs somewhat in the two instances. For when the long arm of a syphon is once filled, the gravitating column of liquid within it instantly acts with its full power in inducing a tendency to the formation of a vacuum in the portion of tube immediately behind it; whereas, the act of inspiration being a gradual effort, the enlargement of the thorax occupies a perceptible interval of time. And therefore, though the partial vacuum formed within the latter may ultimately be capable of raising a column of water to the height of twenty inches, it by no means follows that the derivative force acting on the contents of the large venous trunks is, *at any one moment*, equal to that of a gravitating column of water of this height. On the contrary, as this imperfect vacuum is continually being removed by the influx of additional blood into the thorax, it appears tolerably evident that during an ordinary inspiration this derivative force does not at any one time exceed that of a falling column of water of the same area as the large veins, and three or four inches in height. And if the truth of this remark be admitted, there will then be a tolerably close approximation between the derivative force acting in the living body and that exercised by the syphon in these experiments.

As proving that the absorption and discharge of the stagnant fluid did not depend upon the *direct* action of the syphon, I may mention that the syphon acted so long only as the stream continued to flow through the apparatus. For when that flow ceased the membranous tube was pressed against the orifice of the short arm of the syphon so as to close it; and the long arm then speedily became emptied.

In addition to those already mentioned, there is one other condition which, in the animal body, is found to be essential to the proper circulation of the blood, and more particularly to the due performance of the function of absorption; for it has been clearly proved by the experiments of Hales, and by the experience of all practical anatomists, that in general none other than a thick or viscid fluid can pass through the minute blood-vessels without the occurrence of a very copious effusion. And the truth of this observation is also strikingly exemplified in certain phenomena of disease. As to the manner in which this physical property of the blood assists absorption, it does not appear to me that it exercises any other than an indirect action, viz. that of rendering the blood less apt to escape through the pores of its containing vessels: for as a certain amount of lateral pressure is required to overcome the cohesive force of the particles of blood, and as the impeding causes which occasion that lateral pressure are, in the veins, very few in number, and trivial in their character, it is probable that, in a state of perfect health, little or no effusion takes place through the walls of this portion of the circulating system. To render the chain of evidence more complete, I repeated the same experiments with membranous tubes, observing every particular as before, with the single exception of substituting a viscid fluid, viz. common size, for water; and absorption went on quite as well as when the more mobile liquid was used; there being, moreover, this additional advantage, that the progress of the experiment was less liable to be disturbed by effusion during any slight disorder of the apparatus.

The whole of these considerations will, I trust, be deemed sufficient to establish the principle, *that a stream, while traversing a flaccid membranous tube, can, under certain favourable conditions, exercise an absorbing power*; and if the correctness of this statement be admitted, it will not be difficult to reconcile these views with the knowledge already possessed on the subject of the process of absorption in animals; for as it is fully proved that the act of circulation, or, in other words, the passage of the blood through the minute vessels of the part, is essential to the occurrence of absorption, it now only remains to inquire, 1st, what particular part of the circulating system is the more especial seat of this function, and 2ndly, in what manner the passage of external fluids into the blood-vessels is accomplished.

I may, however, previously remark, that, by thus referring the active absorbing power to the streams of blood, we are at once furnished with a satisfactory explanation of the fact, that the circulation through a part is necessary for the occurrence of an appreciable amount of absorption.

In answer to the first question, I may repeat the statement incidentally made when speaking of the conditions essential to absorption, viz. that this action is confined to the terminating portion of the capillaries and the small veins. In support of this opinion may be mentioned,—

1. The indirect evidence constituted by the facts and arguments adduced in the first part of this memoir, in order to show that an effusion of certain portions of the blood is constantly occurring through the coats of the small arteries and contiguous portion of the capillaries; and if this conclusion be a correct one, it is evident that no *active* absorption can be proceeding in the same.

2. I have attempted to show, by imitative experiments, that every circumstance connected with the arrangement, structure, and relations of the veins, is calculated to favour the absorbing power of the streams of blood by which they are traversed. Thus I found that, with a membranous tube and an ascending stream, absorption could only be obtained by copying, as closely as possible, *every* peculiarity observed in the veins of animals; and while engaged in devising an apparatus which should rudely represent some of the contrivances employed by nature in her most elaborate works, I could not resist the conviction that, if it were possible for man to construct an arborescent system of minute membranous tubes, similar to the veins of animals, the streams traversing which should possess the same physical properties, follow the same converging course, and be in every respect subjected to the same physical conditions as the blood contained within the veins, then the same physical result, viz. the rapid absorption of any external fluid, would most undoubtedly be obtained.

3. Fodera, who watched the process of absorption

under the microscope *, observed the coloured substance to appear first in the most minute venous radicles, and then in the larger veins.

I have before remarked, that the absorbing power of streams is *cæteris paribus* proportioned to their velocity; and, as connected with the point now under consideration, I may refer to the interesting fact, that natural philosophers, from reasoning upon the physical arrangement of the system of blood-vessels, long since concluded that the point where the blood flows with the greatest velocity, is at the commencement of the veins. †

The next question, viz. as to the means by which the passage of fluids into the interior of the blood-vessels is accomplished, involves an examination of the nature of the absorbing power exercised by all rapid streams; and in the following brief explanation of this action, I have endeavoured to limit myself as closely as possible to the relation of such facts as appeared best calculated to render intelligible the process of vascular absorption in animals.

It is well known that a fluid in rapid motion does not press equally in all directions, its lateral being invariably less than its onward pressure; for if those forces were at all equal, every liquid jet, instead of contracting somewhat after escaping from an orifice,

* "Recherches Expérimentales sur l'absorption et l'exhalation," par Michel Fodera, p. 26. Paris, 1824.

† "L'endroit où il (le sang) doit se mouvoir avec le plus de rapidité c'est à l'origine des veines."—Musschenbroek, *Essai de Physique*, t. i. p. 392. Leyden, 1793.

should represent more or less of the appearance of a rapidly diverging cone.

As before mentioned, it has also been proved by the experiments of Venturi and others, that when a rapid stream traverses a short conical tube, the whole surface of that stream possesses the power of drawing into the tube any stagnant fluid with which (by means of a lateral opening) the interior of that tube may communicate; and in repeating these experiments with a strong jet, I have found the same ascent and influx of the external stagnant fluid to occur, whether the communicating glass tube were fastened to the upper, or lower, or lateral, surface of the main pipe.

In explanation of this phenomenon, it may be stated, as a general principle, *that all bodies, while in a state of rapid motion, possess the power of carrying with them the contiguous particles of any surrounding stagnant fluid.* Thus a jet of liquid, or one of gas, or a rapidly revolving wheel, or any projectile, will each speedily cause a current of the surrounding air to flow in the same direction.

I have even found that, on holding the orifice of a glass tube at a right angle to the surface of a strong jet of water, the ascent and discharge into the stream of the liquid into which the other end of the glass tube dipped took place with the same rapidity as when the jet traversed a rigid pipe.* Hence it appears that a stream can exercise an active ab-

* A detailed account of this and some analogous experiments was contained in a Paper lately read before the Royal Society.

sorbing power without necessarily entering any kind of pipe; for it is merely necessary to bring the orifice of the connecting tube in contact with any part of the surface of the stream, inasmuch as the absorbing power exists throughout the whole extent of the moving column. A strong blast of air, directed across the orifice of the tube, caused a similar ascent of the coloured liquid in the other arm.

Now if, instead of an open jet thus made to sweep across the orifices of a great number of tubes held at right angles to it, we suppose a similar current of liquid to flow along a vessel the walls of which are perforated by innumerable small apertures, it can then be readily understood that the stream, in crossing the orifices of all these minute lateral tubes, will exercise the same power of drawing through them any stagnant fluid with which they may communicate externally. In this point of view, the pores situated in the coats of the smaller blood-vessels may be regarded as so many minute short tubes, the internal orifices of which are directed nearly at right angles to the streams of blood, and the external orifices of which are in contact with the various substances absorbed.

The statement that all moving masses possess the power of inducing a corresponding movement of the fluid particles immediately surrounding them being thus capable of direct proof, it now only remains to be shown *that the entrance of an external fluid into the interior of a tube traversed by a rapid stream depends upon a diminution in the amount of pressure acting on the internal surface of that tube.*

The ascent of stagnant liquids observed in the experiments of Venturi has very justly been referred to atmospheric pressure, or, in other words, to diminished pressure *within* the tube traversed by the stream; and that this is the true explanation of the phenomenon is proved by the following among other reasons.

1. To ensure the success of the experiment all the joinings of the apparatus must be perfectly air-tight; otherwise the ascent of the stagnant liquid will be very limited.

2. The same stream which drew up a column of water to the height of twenty inches, raised mercury to the height of one inch and a half only, which elevations bear to each other very nearly the same proportion as the specific gravities of these two liquids.

3. The following experiment, performed by Hanksbee, at the commencement of the last century, is interesting, not only for the clear light which it throws upon the present question, but also from its establishing for this country the credit of the first discovery of this particular property of currents.

A quantity of highly compressed air was made to pass through a pipe, which by means of two lateral branches communicated with the cisterns of as many barometers, one of which was placed at the distance of three feet from the main pipe.

"The result of which was, that this rapid current of air so lessened the pressure of the atmosphere upon the stagnant mercury in the cisterns of the respective barometers, that the mercury was made thereby to descend at least two inches. Nay, that barometer which was three feet distant from the aërial stream was equally affected as the nearer one. And it is further observable, that as the force of the current of air diminished, so the weight of the atmosphere recovered its strength again, and forced the mercury in the barometers to a gradual ascent."* This experiment was undertaken with the view of discovering the cause of the descent of the mercury in barometers during a storm. And I may add, that the few remarks which the author makes upon the probable influence on the animal body of a diminished atmospheric pressure, are, so far as they extend, very much in unison with the physiological principles advocated in this communication.

It is therefore evident, that the entrance of an external fluid into the interior of a porous tube traversed by a rapid stream, is a consequence of the pressure then acting on the internal surface of that tube being less than that of the surrounding medium.

When the tube is exposed to the air, and a quantity of this gaseous fluid is absorbed, the pressure of the atmosphere is evidently the sole cause of the phenomenon; but when liquids are absorbed, the weight of the external stagnant column co-operates with that of the atmosphere in effecting absorption.

In the animal body, this external pressure—the *immediate* cause of absorption — varies much in

* "Physico-Mechanical Experiments," pp. 114, 115. By F. Hauksbee, F.R.S. Second edition. London, 1719.

different parts, both as to its degree, and also as to the nature of the particular forces constituting it.

Thus in the lungs, the weight of the atmosphere is the only force that can act on the exterior of those minute blood-vessels through which absorption is known to occur with extreme rapidity; whereas the whole contents of the abdomen are, in addition to being subjected to the action of the ordinary causes of external pressure, forcibly compressed by the diaphragm and abdominal muscles. By the contractions of the alimentary canal, the nutritious matters are, moreover, forced against the walls of the blood-vessels ramifying upon the intestinal coats.

This latter fact—viz., that in that particular part of the body where the absorption of food is effected, there exists throughout the animated creation an express contrivance for increasing the pressure acting on the exterior of the blood-vessels— does appear to me to constitute a very powerful argument in support of this view of the nature of the absorbing process. And when, in the treatment of disease, a more active absorption is desirable, experience has shown that there is no more effectual mode of accomplishing this object than by increasing the external pressure in the affected part. It is, of course, requisite that the external force applied should never exceed a moderate amount; otherwise the circulation through the part, and with it all absorption, would be totally arrested; whereas a more gentle support not only facilitates absorption *directly*, by forcing the surrounding fluids into the interior of the blood-vessels, but, by diminishing the diameter of the latter, and thus increasing the velocity of the currents of blood, it also adds *indirectly* to their absorbing power.

I have made no mention of the manner in which absorption might be supposed to be effected by the lacteals and lymphatics, because it appears to me very doubtful whether those vessels really possess any *active* absorbing power of their own. On the contrary, the information already possessed on the subject of absorption, the intimate connection shown to exist between the rapidity of the circulation of the blood and the activity of the absorbing process, the dependence of the latter on the former action, and the absence of any adequate mechanism in the so-called absorbent vessels, all tend to invest with probability the opinion—which was, I believe, first advanced by my friend Mr. Fenwick*—viz., that the substances contained in these vessels are derived from the adjacent blood-vessels by a process of effusion analogous to secretion.

It might to some appear improbable, that in a system of continuous tubes like the blood-vessels, through the walls of which, in the earlier part of their course, effusion has been shown to occur, the opposite process of absorption should nevertheless be enabled to proceed throughout the rest of their extent. To meet this difficulty, I may briefly relate three experiments—one performed with a rigid, another with an elastic and yielding, and the third with a membranous tube—in order to show that,

* "Medical Gazette," July 21st, 1843, vol. xxxii. p. 605.

when a stream encounters an obstacle in the middle portion of a tube, effusion necessarily occurs through any lateral openings situated behind the impediment, while absorption will, in accordance with the principle illustrated by one of the experiments to which I have referred, proceed with increased rapidity through the apertures placed on the other side of the obstacle, viz., nearer to the discharging orifice.

Exp. 3. A leaden pipe, a yard long, and half an inch in diameter—the central part of which had previously been much curved—was fastened horizontally to a reservoir, and two small apertures were made on its upper surface at a short distance from either end of the curved portion of the tube. On passing a stream of water through it, the impediments, constituted by the existence of these lateral curves, caused a small jet to escape from the aperture placed behind the latter, while a rapid absorption of air, or of any other stagnant fluid with which it communicated, took place through the opening situated nearer to the discharging orifice of the pipe.

Exp. 4. A piece of the aorta of the horse, eight inches in length, was fastened horizontally to the reservoir, and two bent glass tubes, one arm of which dipped into a coloured liquid, were inserted into two of its lateral branches situated at a distance of four inches from each other, all the other lateral openings being carefully closed. The central portion of the pipe was now grasped at a point equally distant from the insertion of both glass tubes, and its calibre there considerably diminished, so that the stream would in the first instance pass from the wide to the narrow portion of a conical tube, and subsequently from the narrow to the wide part of a similar tube. Under these circumstances, a copious effusion occurred through the glass tube communicating with the first portion of the pipe, and an active absorption through that leading to its second division.

Exp. 5. The perforated membranous tube used with the apparatus described under Experiment 2, being held horizontally in the open air, and slightly pressed at one point, effusion occurred through the lateral apertures behind that point, while numerous globules of air entered those situated nearer to the escaping jet.

It will, I trust, now be considered as proved, that the active power employed in the animal body for the performance of absorption resides in the currents of blood which incessantly traverse the veins and terminating portion of the capillaries. This opinion, like that of Magendie, rests upon the fact of the permeability or porosity of the walls of the smaller blood-vessels; but it differs from his in withdrawing the substances placed in contact with those pores from the sole control of powers with which we are not well acquainted, and in substituting for the latter the more general and intelligible cause of fluid motion; viz., unequal pressure.

I agree with Sir D. Barry in thinking that the relative vacuum formed within the thorax during the act of inspiration, greatly assists the process of absorption. But I contend that it does so *indirectly* and *mediately;* viz., by increasing the rapidity, and facilitating the passage of the streams of blood traversing the veins.

As giving a concise view of the general action of the causes producing effusion and absorption, it may be stated that effusion is promoted, 1st, *directly,* by whatever *increases* the amount of pressure acting on the *internal* surface of the blood-vessels; and 2ndly, *indirectly,* by whatever *diminishes* the pressure acting on their *exterior:* while absorption is rendered more active, 1st, by whatever *directly increases* the amount of *external* pressure; and 2ndly, by whatever increases the rapidity of the currents of blood; and thus *diminishes* the pressure acting on the *internal* surface of the absorbing blood-vessels.

Part III.

BEING AN ATTEMPT TO INQUIRE HOW FAR THE ENTRANCE OF CERTAIN GASES INTO, AND THE DISCHARGE OF OTHERS FROM, THE INTERIOR OF THE BLOOD-VESSELS, MAY BE ACCOUNTED FOR ON THE GENERAL PRINCIPLES OF EFFUSION AND ABSORPTION.

It now only remains to inquire how far the same views are applicable to the explanation of those functions in animals which consist in the extrication and discharge of certain gases from, and the absorption of others into, the mass of circulating blood. Here the doctrine of capillary attraction is confessed to be incapable of explaining the phenomena*: they are therefore generally referred to the mutual penetrability of gases.

That the extrication of carbonic acid in the lungs is materially facilitated by this property of diffusion, I can readily believe; but are we to suppose that this discharge of carbonic acid from the blood occurs equally in *every part of the pulmonary vessels*, and that the absorption of oxygen in like manner takes place with equal activity in the minute arteries and veins, and throughout the whole extent of the capillaries of the lung? There are many recorded observations which militate strongly against such a supposition. And as many of these phenomena are perfectly explicable by the general principles of effusion and absorption, I may, perhaps, be excused for now briefly noticing some of the more important of them. It was shown by Lower, not long after the discovery of the circulation, that the change from venous to arterial blood takes place during the passage of the former fluid through the small vessels of the lungs. Subsequent experiments have proved that this change consists essentially in the discharge of carbonic acid from, and the absorption of oxygen into, the mass of blood. And as the blood circulating through the lungs does not present the bright red colour of arterial blood till it has entered the small pulmonary veins, this circumstance alone justifies the presumption that the absorption of oxygen by the blood is effected in this part of its course.

* Magendie, "Journal," t. i. p. 16.

The property of mutual diffusion possessed by gases, is useful, not only as facilitating the discharge of carbonic acid gas through the lining membranes of the lung, but also from its enabling us to explain why that discharge is not general throughout the body, and why it only takes place on a free surface; where the external pressure is inconsiderable, and where the surrounding atmosphere presents a species of vacuum into which the imprisoned and compressed gases may freely expand. But it does not throw any light upon the means by which gases are *absorbed* into the blood. And I shall now mention some reasons for thinking that the absorption of gases is effected in the same manner as that of liquids; viz., by a preponderance of the pressure acting on the exterior of the absorbing blood-vessels.

1. That the absorption of oxygen in the lungs takes place in the terminating portion of the capillaries and the small pulmonary veins, is, to say the least, rendered highly probable by the above-mentioned observation of Lower.

2. The general absorbing power of the healthy lung is extremely active; so that any poisonous substance brought in contact with its lining membrane produces its effect upon the system almost instantaneously.

3. Atmospheric air, or any other gas injected into the cellular tissue of the body, is, if the quantity be moderate, speedily absorbed.

4. It is fully proved that streams of liquid possess the power of absorbing, through the lateral apertures of the containing tube, any gaseous fluids that may

be in contact with the exterior of the latter. I have also found that this absorption will occur through an intervening layer of animal membrane.

Since, then, all other rapid streams, while traversing porous tubes, possess the power of absorbing any external contiguous gases, since that power is shown to be possessed by the streams of blood passing through the systemic blood-vessels, and since the general absorbing power of the pulmonary blood-currents is known to be extremely active, it appears to me impossible to resist the conclusion, that the entrance of gases into the mass of blood circulating through the lungs takes place in the same part of the blood-vessels, and is effected in the same manner, as the absorption of liquids.

This view is moreover supported by some experiments by Leroy d'Etiolles, and related by him in Magendie's Journal.* He found that on causing animals to breathe highly compressed air, and thus increasing the external pressure acting on the blood-vessels of the lung, the absorption of that air was so rapid, that the whole mass of blood not unfrequently became quite frothy.

And the whole of these considerations also tend to prove the correctness of the opinion in part entertained by Sir H. Davy†; viz., that the atmospheric air is, in the lungs, absorbed as such (for we know of no power by which the oxygen could be taken into the blood-vessels and the nitrogen rejected); that the

* "Journal de Physiologie," t. viii. pp. 106 and 109.

† "Researches concerning the Nitrous Oxide." London, 1800 pp. 429, 447, 449, &c.

oxygen of the absorbed air combines with certain portions of the blood during the systemic circulation, and that the residual nitrogen is, with the carbonic acid, discharged through the walls of the exhaling portion of the pulmonary vessels.

It is known that the opposite change from arterial to venous blood depends upon the presence of carbonie acid in the latter fluid; and it is generally believed that this change is effected in the systemic capillaries and minute veins, by the absorption of various products resulting from the decomposition of the tissues. Among other matters carbonic acid is, of course, copiously generated, and by its absorption the change of colour is produced. In like manner, when the main artery of a limb is tied, the blood which enters the trunk below the ligature, and which has necessarily passed through minute anastmosing branches, is immediately found to possess the colour of venous blood. Now this blood has evidently been placed under nearly the same physical conditions as the blood contained in the veins; for to arrive at the lower portion of the main artery, it must have traversed two systems of arborescent tubes; in the first of which the streams diverge, and in the second converge.

Those streams, therefore, which flow in the same course as the currents contained within the veins, exercise the same property of absorption; whence the change of colour resulting from the entrance into the blood of a quantity of carbonic acid.

It thus appears that while the absorbing blood-vessels of the lung take in atmospheric air, those distributed throughout the rest of the system receive carbonic acid; which, with that generated in the mass of blood itself, escapes from the exhalant vessels of the lungs.

Physiologists and natural philosophers have long supposed that many of the purposes served in the animal economy by the circulation of the blood are accomplished by the operation of ordinary hydrodynamic principles.

In the preceding remarks I have endeavoured, through the medium of those principles, to establish an intimate connection between certain important functions in animals and the great discovery of Harvey, viz., the *incessant motion of the blood.* In the course of this attempt I may occasionally appear to have diverged somewhat from my more immediate subject; but these slight digressions, if they should be considered such, may perhaps be pardoned, inasmuch as they constitute an imperfection which must be common to all who seek for a solution of the mysteries of organic life in the simpler, and not less beautiful, laws of inanimate matter.

ON THE

NATURE AND PRINCIPLES OF TREATMENT OF INFLAMMATION,

AND THE

ALLIED DISORDERS OF THE CIRCULATION.

(From the LONDON MEDICAL GAZETTE, 1846–7.)

ON no subject in the whole range of medical science has more been written than on inflammation: a fact sufficiently indicative both of the importance and difficulty of its study. Nor can any investigations yet published be said to have so far settled the various questions involved in the consideration of the precise nature of this disease, as to preclude others from entering upon the same field of inquiry. Indeed, most of the writers upon inflammation seem, in some measure, to have evaded the discussion of the great point, as to its essential nature, and have contented themselves with describing the order of production of its symptoms and effects. The professed definitions of it which I have met with, have generally been of two kinds: either an enumeration of its phenomena, varying in length from the classical brevity of Celsus to a tedious diffuseness which filled more than one page, or some dogma which appealed rather to the faith than to the reason of the inquirer. Those more rational doctrines, in which it has recently been endeavoured to base the elucidation of its pathology upon the disordered condition of the circulation in the affected part, will, of course, be hereafter considered in detail. But before stating the experiments and reasoning which appear to me to establish certain views in this department of the pathology of the circulation, I may, perhaps, be permitted to allude to a circumstance which has, in my opinion, prevented those doctrines, though ably advocated, from conducting to any satisfactory and final solution of the difficulty: and that circumstance is, the paucity and indirectness of the facts on which they rest.

In order to test the accuracy of this statement, let any one examine for himself the different works on inflammation, and scrutinise and classify the facts adduced in support of the various views therein advocated. And with the exception of those long-observed phenomena which, though recorded for centuries, led to no extension of our actual knowledge of the disease, these facts will be found to consist of experimental observations upon the lower animals. It is exclusively from the latter that the more precise information which we now possess on the subject has been derived; and from them also have originated all the modern ideas as to the essential nature of inflammation and its allied morbid conditions. The importance of a clear conception of the force and pertinency of these facts, and of the extent to which the resulting conclusions may be applied towards the elucidation and settlement of the general question, will therefore be sufficiently obvious.

These experiments may be conveniently considered under two heads. In the first division we have those performed by Hunter himself upon some of the higher animals; in the second group may be comprised all those numerous microscopical observations upon the transparent tissues of various reptiles and of certain of the higher animals, in which the successive phenomena presented by a part artificially inflamed, have been carefully watched, and minutely described, by Wilson Philip, Hastings, Gendrin, and a host of observers.

Now it can, I think, be shown that all these experiments and observations, though most valuable from the light which they have cast upon the mode of production of certain of the symptoms, and the order of development of the effects of inflammation, do not, if fairly considered, conduct the unprejudiced mind to any direct and positive conclusion as to the essential nature of the disease. Before endeavouring to establish this point by a brief review of Hunter's experiments, let me utterly disclaim all idea of attempting to detract from his well-earned fame. On the contrary, as the first successful cultivator of experimental pathology, he has ever been a peculiar object of my veneration: and it will, if I mistake not, be in after ages considered not the least brilliant achievement of human genius that it furnished this great man with sagacity to perceive the inadequacy of mere *observation* as an instrument for pathological discovery, and with ingenuity and boldness to *combine with it* the more subtle and far-reaching agency of *experiment*. In acting thus, it is true that he did but follow out, not only the general principles of the Baconian philosophy, but the suggestions made almost on this very point by that wonderfully gifted man. The gratitude and respect of posterity are, however, not the less due to him who actually effected the first step towards the elevation of medicine by rendering its most important branch an experimental science.

The only experiments of Hunter which can be considered as calculated to throw a direct light upon the nature of inflammation, are the two following: —1st. That of freezing the ear of a rabbit; by which he proved that the vessels of an inflamed part are much enlarged, contain more than their natural quantity of blood, and retain that increased calibre for some time after the withdrawal of the exciting cause. 2ndly. That of inflaming the vagina of an ass; by means of which he discovered the beautiful law, that the temperature of an inflamed part does not rise above that of the central organs of the body. The facts thus ascertained, and the additional experiments which he instituted, relative to the contractility of the arteries, and the peculiarities of adhesive union and growth, are confessedly important, original, useful in enabling us to understand the manner in which certain effects of the disease are produced, and in some respects deeply interesting, as possibly constituting the germs of more important, discoveries. But, while freely admitting all this, I defy the most zealous Hunterian to deduce from them a clear and satisfactory definition of inflammation.

The experimental observations of Thomson,

Philip, and others, next claim our attention. These, even more than those of Hunter, have served as the chief support of all the modern views on the pathology of inflammation. That they have supplied a number of very interesting and important facts, by which we have been enabled to understand the order of the phenomena which occur in a part inflamed by the application of a local irritant, no one can deny. Where, formerly, all was vain conjecture, we have now, through them, obtained a minute and well authenticated history of the successive changes which occur in a part thus affected. For it may be assumed that in conjunctivitis following the lodgment of a foreign body on the eye, or in any other case of inflammation consequent on the application of a local irritant, the course of events is, in the human body, analogous to that witnessed under the microscope in the web of a frog's foot, or in the mesentery of the mouse or rabbit. But I cannot perceive how this information is to suggest the immediate cause, or explain the nature of idiopathic inflammation. Nor am I satisfied that the most minute observation of its effects will, in this or any other case, lead to the detection, or elucidate the operation, of the immediate cause of a disease. And, in the present instance, it must be confessed that, so far from having settled the discussion as to the essential nature of inflammation, these microscopical observations, by introducing into the consideration of a subject already sufficiently complicated, innumerable obscure questions connected with the physiology and pathology of the blood, have added much to the difficulty of reducing chaotic mixture to something like the harmony and simplicity of truth.

I have now endeavoured to show that all these experiments, though most useful and valuable so far as they extend, nevertheless fail to impress the mind with any satisfactory and definite opinion as to the nature of the particular pathological condition essentially constituting inflammation. In order to attain that knowledge, additional facts are required, which shall exhibit in a clearer light than has yet been accomplished the operation of each of the two great causes of disordered circulation. And it is only by the aid of a body of experiments, undertaken for that object, and tolerably conclusive in their results, that I can indulge in the hope of being enabled to advance the settlement of this long-agitated question.

The great confusion which now surrounds the subject of inflammation, has apparently arisen, not more from its intrinsic difficulties than from the clumsy, ill-arranged, and disorderly manner in which its study has been conducted. Instead of resolving into separate questions the numerous considerations which spring from an observation of its attendant phenomena, and then examining each singly, we find writers losing themselves, and bewildering their readers, by attempting to grasp, and master at once, a host of problems, among which are some of the most important, the most extensive, and the most difficult in the whole science of life. Thus, in most treatises on the pathology of this disease, we find heaped together in one confused mass, dissertations and conjectures of various length, according to the particular views of the author, upon each of the following, in addition to other less important topics —viz. the reciprocal influence of the different parts of the nervous system upon the circulation of the blood, and of the circulation upon the action of the nerves; the peculiar functions of the ganglionic nervous system; the chemical composition, and minute anatomical structure of the blood in general, and of that in the inflamed part in particular; the mechanism of the circulation, and more especially the nature of the forces carrying the blood through the capillaries; the physical, vital, and, according to some, electro-vital properties of the latter vessels; the mode of operation of the self-coagulating and self-organising principle of the blood; the order of development and minute peculiarities of the phenomena thus induced; and the nature, origin, and action of the "*specific*," or unknown, causes which so frequently and so powerfully modify those effects.

Now an examination of some of these points certainly constitutes an essential preliminary to the study of the pathology of inflammation, but they need not be continually introduced in the discussion of the greater question; and there are others, perhaps a majority of them, which the present imperfect state of our knowledge will not allow us satisfactorily to decide, and which a spirit of philosophical prudence would therefore rather reserve for future investigation.

Leaving, then, for another opportunity, or for other persons, the consideration of these and various other interesting and important matters connected with general physiology and pathology, let me briefly state the manner in which I propose to conduct this inquiry. For it seems to me that the only sure way of progressing in this, or any other department of pathology, is to lay down and strictly adhere to a clear, well-defined plan of procedure.

In all the different forms of inflammation, however modified its effects, however varied its causation, the same term is universally applied to denote the general nature of the disease. Whether, in any particular case, it be regarded as adhesive, suppurative, erysipelatous, syphilitic, rheumatic, scrofulous, acute, or chronic; in short, whatever may be the epithet joined with it to express some peculiarity in its origin, intensity, or effects, the same essential pathological condition is always admitted to be present. It has further been established by the latest inquirers, that certain physical phenomena invariably accompany it as immediate effects, and constitute the only satisfactory proofs of its existence. Now, the task on which I am about to enter is the elucidation of the nature of this constant pathological condition, and the explanation of the manner in which it is itself produced, and of its mode of action in causing those definite effects which so generally result from its continuance. And it is solely to the illustration of what I may be allowed to term the mechanism of inflammation that my facts and arguments will now be directed. The peculiarities of action of those subtle and ill-understood causes which induce the varieties met with in its *secondary* effects, must remain for the most part unintelligible till such time as the accumulation of a mass of fresh facts shall enable us to deduce laws capable of dispelling the darkness and mystery in which they are now enveloped.

Part II.

OF THE HEALTHY FUNCTIONS OF THE MINUTE BLOOD-VESSELS.

As it is utterly impossible to form any correct idea of the nature of a morbid action without having first thoroughly understood the uses served in their healthy state by the particular structures affected, it is unnecessary to apologise for the introduction, in this place, for a few remarks on the physiology of the circulation; and as the minute blood-vessels are universally admitted to be the seat of the important disorders now under consideration, we cannot satisfactorily engage in the pathological inquiry without first endeavouring to determine the nature of their healthy functions, and, as far as possible, the means by which those actions are accomplished. It is, perhaps, in the present advanced state of physiology, scarcely necessary to combat the proposition so long and so tenaciously maintained, that the arteries and capillaries contribute some active share towards the motion of the blood—the power of the heart being supposed to be inadequate to this task. I may, however, remark that it is as impossible to demonstrate the insufficiency of the heart on the one hand as it is on the other to exhibit in any of the vessels of the circulating apparatus an auxiliary source of power. But while admitting that the propulsion and distribution of the blood are mechanical processes, physiologists seem, by common consent, to have referred to certain powers assumed to exist in the capillary blood-vessels, the causation of all those important functions which are evidently more or less intimately connected with the blood's circulation.

Now, why the chain of connection between this motion of the blood as a cause, and the production of these actions as effects, should be so abruptly broken by the interposition of a mysterious membrane operating by laws which we cannot understand, inasmuch as they are totally different from those regulating the interchange of fluids through membrane, is a question which I have never been able to answer to my own satisfaction. Nor can I understand why mechanism should be supposed to cease with the mere transmission of the blood. On the contrary, it would seem much more consonant with our general experience of the beautiful simplicity of Nature's arrangements to suppose that by some skilful adaptation, some simple contrivance, the force imparted to the mass of blood by the heart's action, existing with that blood in every minute vessel of the body, and thus constituting an infinitely graduated, ubiquitous, and unceasing power, is the immediate cause of many of those actions which have hitherto been ascribed to occult and unintelligible agencies.

In a former communication to this Journal (June and July 1844), I endeavoured, by numerous physical and physiological facts and arguments, to establish the following law, viz. that "all those functions which involve either the discharge through the coats of the minute blood-vessels of certain matters previously present in the blood, or the entrance of various external substances into the mass of circulating fluid, are dependent upon a preponderance, in one or other direction, of the forces acting on either surface of those vessels." It follows, therefore, as immediate consequences of this law, that *effusion,* or the *outward* passage of fluids through the capillary membrane is promoted, 1st, *directly* by whatever increases the amount of pressure acting on the *internal* surface of the blood-vessels; and 2ndly, *indirectly* by whatever *diminishes* the pressure acting on their *exterior.* While *absorption,* or the *inward* passage of fluids through the same porous structure is rendered more active, 1st, by whatever *directly increases* the amount of *external* pressure; and 2ndly, by whatever increases the rapidity of the currents of blood, and thus *diminishes* the pressure acting on the *internal* surface of those blood-vessels which are subservient to this function. In assigning to the minute arterial twigs and contiguous capillaries, a certain, constant, but moderate, amount of *effusion* as their natural and specific use in the animal economy*, and in referring to the

* Though compelled to speak of the function of the arterial, as distinguished from that of the venous capillaries, I am anxious to have it distinctly understood as my opinion, that the *coats of these*

incipient venous radicles the opposite and equally important action of *absorption*, I mentioned at some length the physical and anatomical facts which support these views. As regards the accomplishment of the first action, it is, therefore, on the present occasion, only necessary for me to state, that the obstacles to the free passage of the arterial blood cause that fluid, when entering the capillaries, to exert a certain amount of lateral pressure, by means of which its albuminous portion is continually, though slowly, exuding for the purposes of nutrition.

While the streams of blood, having once entered the most contracted point of the capillary blood-vessels, so far from encountering causes of impediment, are facilitated in their course by the most perfect mechanical arrangement of the sanguiferous tubes, and consequently, like all other freely moving currents, then begin to exercise a power of lateral draught, and thus induce that preponderance of the external pressure which causes the act of absorption.

But it is impossible to advance a step further in the study of the physiology or pathology of the circulation until the term "capillaries" is clearly defined, and some attempt is made to confine within reasonable bounds their healthy powers and uses. In an anatomical point of view, many eminent men seem to think that the term "capillaries" should be restricted to those cylindrical intermediate tubes

vessels take no part whatever in the causation of either process; the active power, which induces both effusion and absorption, being, in the healthy state, wholly derived from the columns of blood contained within those vessels.

which connect the two great systems of divergent and convergent blood-vessels. And if we admit the correctness of the prevailing opinion, that all the great functions of the circulation, such as secretion, nutrition, and absorption, are in some incomprehensible manner performed by these highly endowed tubules, and that the contiguous arteries and veins, and, in fact, all the different parts of the circulating system, are provided for the sole purpose of supplying them with blood, it may then be convenient to retain this exclusive application of the term. But both the anatomical and physiological reasons in favour of the maintenance of this distinction would seem to be destroyed by the fact, that in certain tissues of the body some of those functions do proceed, and inflammation and other morbid actions do occur, although no such intermediate cylindrical vessels can be shown to exist. The opinion has, in all probability, arisen from a too hasty application to the whole body of the results furnished by a microscopical examination of the blood's course through the lungs, where, for a specific purpose, the extent of the intermediate vessels is greatly increased. And as I am not aware of any satisfactory reasons for supposing that these intermediate vessels possess functions different from those of the contiguous venous and arterial ramifications; and as the latter, and more especially the adjacent arterial twigs, are, equally with the former vessels, the seat of those disorders of the circulation which are now about to be considered, I shall use the term "capillary" in its literal sense as synonymous with "minute."

In concluding this brief recapitulation of the views contained in my former paper, it only remains for me to add, that as the relative facilities afforded for the passage of the blood through the minute vessels of different organs and structures must necessarily vary with the anatomical arrangement of those vessels, so will the activity, and even the nature, of these functions which are connected with the amount of lateral pressure of the blood-currents be in the same proportion affected. In a secreting structure, where effusion is continually occurring, the internal pressure will preponderate in the intermediate vessels as completely as in the minute diverging ones: while in a vascular arrangement, like that of the lung, it appears to me very certain that the cylindrical vessels possess an absorbing power not inferior to that of the adjacent veins. It is also, from the same reasoning, evident that a vessel which, in a healthy state, absorbs, will, on the application of an obstruction to the blood's passage through it, lose that power, and take on the opposite action—effusion. The same portion of capillary tube may, therefore, at different times, and under opposite conditions, be an absorbing and an effusing vessel.

Part III.

OF THE OPINIONS HITHERTO HELD AS TO THE ESSENTIAL NATURE OF INFLAMMATION.

Having thus briefly recapitulated the views which I have been led to entertain as to the healthy actions of the minute blood-vessels, there remains but one additional topic to be noticed before entering upon an examination of the great question selected for the present inquiry. And, however delicate and difficult the task, I must not be deterred by any feelings of timidity or respect for individuals, from concisely stating, and candidly criticising, the prevalent opinions on the subject. In *all* scientific investigations, the love of truth should be held paramount to every other consideration. But in the examination of questions connected with *medical* science, and particularly in the study of an important and extensive disease like inflammation, where the interests of humanity are so evidently and immediately promoted by the advancement of our knowledge, an undue reverence for the opinions of others would indeed be an unpardonable weakness.

It is not my intention, were it in my power, to attempt any lengthened review of the numerous doctrines which have successively been presented to, and for a time adopted by, the profession. Such a display of erudition would in this, as in many other cases, be much more curious than instructive; for, as far as my limited observation has enabled me to judge, the settlement of a difficult and long-agitated question is not in general much facilitated by an extended series of quotations. My remarks will therefore chiefly bear upon those views which, either from their present popularity, or from their resemblance or antagonism to my own, could not very well be passed over in silence.

Were it now necessary to insist upon, not merely the *study*, but the *advancement* of physiology, as an indispensable preliminary to the successful cultivation of pathological science, no stronger argument could be presented than an appeal to the history of the various doctrines which have at different periods been promulgated as to the nature of inflammation. For we find each to have been based upon certain peculiar views of the physiology of the circulation, none of which seem to have possessed sufficient solidity to withstand the attacks of more recent inquirers; and the consequence has been, the gradual downfall of the pathological doctrines which were based upon erroneous or obscure views of the natural actions of the body.

The first author to whom I shall allude is Boerhaave, whose ideas on this subject may, by some, be considered to approximate very closely to those which I have adopted. But a slight examination of his writings will suffice to show that, beyond the fact of our mutually recognising a mechanical obstruction as the universal concomitant and cause of inflammation, my views of the essential nature of this disease and of the manner in which it operates in the production of its effects, are very different from those taught by that sagacious and accomplished physician.

Cullen's doctrine, of a spasm of the extreme vessels, which, as an occasional *predisposing* or *exciting* cause of inflammation, must, I think, be to a certain extent adopted, will be more conveniently considered in a subsequent part of this communication.

The celebrated work of John Hunter, which, even to this day, influences the opinions of many eminent writers on inflammation, and which must ever be studied with respect and diligence as embodying the matured views of a most able and experienced man, does not, so far at least as I can judge, throw any direct light on the nature of the disease. His practical precepts are doubtless most excellent, and many of the pathological principles which he deduced from his careful and prolonged observation of disease evince the deepest reflection and the highest powers of generalisation. But his views, both of the healthy and diseased actions of the body, are so deeply tinged with the mysticism of the vitalists, that their unlimited adoption would be equivalent to a total prohibition of all further progress in this important department of pathology. I shall only add that, though Hunter is generally considered as adverse to the idea of *obstruction* constituting the essential cause of inflammation, the passage on which this conclusion rests is in itself so ambiguous, and so much at variance with the remarks immediately following it, that the authority of his name may just as fairly be placed on one side of the question as on the other.

The signal failure of Boerhaave's attempt to found a mechanical doctrine of inflammation seems to have deterred modern pathologists from ever directing their thoughts to the possibility of its being, in all its essential characteristics, a purely physical disorder. They have consequently, in alluding to the question of its nature, contented themselves with describing as minutely as possible the changes which are observed to take place in an inflamed part, the production of those changes being of course referred to nervous, or vital, or, in other words, to some unknown agency. It is not, therefore, surprising that the discussions which occupy so prominent a place in the modern history of inflammation should have reference rather to the correctness of some disputed observation, or the adjustment of some incidental and secondary question, than to the establishment of a great principle explanatory of the nature, causation, and consequences of this disorder of the circulation. We accordingly find that the investigations of Thomson, Philip, Hastings, and others, are chiefly directed to the settlement of the dispute as to whether the action of the vessels is inordinately increased or diminished in the inflamed part. It is not always very easy to understand the precise meaning intended to be expressed by the term *action;* but so far as relates to the establishment of the fact of the enlargement of the minute blood-vessels, and the gradual retardation and ultimate stagnation of the blood contained within them, the microscopical observations of these gentlemen are sufficiently conclusive.

Dr. C. J. B. Williams, in some lectures which appeared in the "Medical Gazette" during the year 1841, and the substance of which is incorporated in his recent publication on the Principles of Medicine, has certainly treated this interesting and important subject in a much more rational spirit than, with one exception, any preceding writer. His definition of inflammation is, however, liable to the same objection which I have urged against those of other modern pathologists, viz. that *it merely describes certain phenomena of the disease*, without imparting to the mind of the reader any definite idea of its real nature; for he defines inflammation as "local hyperæmia in a part; the motion of that blood being partly increased and partly diminished." And beyond the fact of its drawing a distinction between the rate of motion of the blood contained in the part actually inflamed, and that circulating in the adjacent capillaries, I must confess my inability to perceive in this definition any more precise information as to the essential nature of the disease than is to be found in that of Celsus.

The writer who has, in my opinion, exhibited the greatest ability in his examination of this subject, is Mr. J. W. Earle. His papers, published in the "Medical Gazette," during the year 1835, not only evince great sagacity and high powers of reasoning, but also show their author to have been animated by a sincere love of truth. On one or two important points he has suggested views almost identical with those which have been forced upon me by my own reflection and researches. But his adoption of

Wedemeyer's idea, that the capillaries are membraneless canals, mere grooves or channels in the parenchyma, without any proper investing coat; his inability to adduce any direct and positive facts in support of his opinion, and his retention of, what I must conceive to be, erroneous and obscure views of the physiology of the circulation, would probably, for an indefinite period, have prevented his explanation from receiving the attention which it merits. If the correctness of the principle which I am about to endeavour to establish should ever be generally admitted, whatever credit may be attached to a partial anticipation of the doctrine is certainly, as far as I know, due to Mr. Earle. And I have the more pleasure in admitting this priority in the conception of the leading idea, inasmuch as that gentleman is personally unknown to me, and our views are, in almost every other particular, diametrically opposite.

Part IV.

OF THE LAWS REGULATING THE EFFECTS OF OBSTRUCTED CAPILLARY CIRCULATION, AS DEDUCED FROM A COURSE OF EXPERIMENTS ON THE KIDNEY.

It has always appeared to me an extraordinary circumstance, that, while every theory of inflammation which has appeared since the discovery of the circulation more or less explicitly recognises the existence of some unnatural obstruction to the blood's passage through the minute vessels of the affected part, no attempts have been made to determine, by actual experiment, the degree of connection between that disorder of the circulation and the chain of pathological phenomena of which it is the invariable concomitant. We do indeed find that so long since as the time of Lower it was known that an obstruction to the flow of blood through the large venous trunks caused the effusion of its more aqueous portion into any free spaces in the parts below. But, with the exception of isolated observations of this nature, nothing seems to have been effected towards the elucidation, by direct experimental evidence, of the morbid changes induced, in a healthy part or organ, by the existence of a local impediment to the circulation.

And before relating the facts which will constitute the chief support of the following views on the nature of inflammation, it may not be altogether useless or uninteresting to give here a brief account of the manner in which I became gradually involved in the investigation of this subject.

In the autumn of 1841, being then engaged in studying the nature of granular disease of the kidney, and feeling disposed to consider it as essentially congestive or inflammatory in its origin, it occurred to me that the most ready and satisfactory method of deciding the question would be, to ascertain by experiment how far similar phenomena could be induced by the artificial production of simple nephritis. And, "from reflecting on the great obstruction to the circulation through the minute vessels of an inflamed part, I was led to imagine that, by preventing the return of blood from the kidney in one of the lower animals, and taking care not to injure the artery in the experiment, a condition of the organ similar to that present in acute nephritis would be produced."* The result of one or two trials proved this expectation to have been well founded; and, thus encouraged, I proceeded, in the course of the following summer, to extend my observations, and to vary the conditions of the experiment. The facts thus obtained, appearing sufficiently numerous and decisive to justify me in attempting to discard the generally received opinions on the subject, were embodied in a paper on the nature of inflammation; but the publication of these views has, from a variety of causes, been delayed till the present moment. The experiments themselves, and the conclusions to which they directly led, were, however, through the kindness of Dr. Marshall Hall, presented to the Royal Medical and Chirurgical Society, in February 1843, and published in the next volume of that Society's Transactions. And, on the whole, this delay has not been without some advantage. For the intervening period has not only

* An Inquiry into the Nature of Granular Disease of the Kidney, p. 30, 1842. This little brochure will be found to contain, in a conjectural form, most of the physiological and pathological principles embodied in this communication. There is, however, an important error in it which I am anxious to correct. It arose from my confusion of the lobules visible on the surface of the kidney with the proper Malpighian bodies, since described by Mr. Bowman. But, as my reasoning was evidently intended to apply to the former, it becomes rather a verbal error than one of fact.

allowed me to satisfy myself, by deliberate reflection, of the accuracy of my original impressions, but has also enabled me to investigate some important points in the physiology of the circulation, and thus, I trust, given greater clearness and comprehensiveness to my views on the local derangements of that great instrument of animal life.

It will thus be seen that these researches were not, in the first instance, directed to the attainment of any higher object than the settlement of some points connected with the morbid appearances and effects of nephritis. And it was their success in illustrating the mode of production of certain phenomena of this particular affection which encouraged me to extend my observations, in the hope of obtaining results applicable to the elucidation of the general subject of inflammation. Another important inducement to persevere in this extended inquiry arose from the conviction that no other organ in the body presents equal facilities with the kidney for an experimental investigation of this nature. In any of the lower animals, this gland, particularly that of the left side, can be readily reached and exposed by an incision in the loins, passing between the lumbar and abdominal muscles. And, as its connections with the surrounding structures are very slight, it can, if required, be drawn out through the wound, its vessels and duct isolated, and, if necessary, secured by ligature; and the organ then returned without the infliction of any material injury to it or any other vital structure. Then its blood-vessels are so arranged that, while both vein and artery are equally accessible, the whole of the blood passing into, and returning from, the gland, must traverse these trunks; and consequently, by acting on one or other of them, we have the circulation through the organ completely under command. And availing myself, to the fullest extent, of the advantages thus offered, I have not only studied the effects of obstructed circulation as induced by a partial or complete occlusion of the renal vein, but have also, in an organ healthy and untouched, caused phenomena identical with those of acute inflammation, by obstructing the abdominal aorta *below* the origin of the renal arteries, and at the same time tying the vessels of the left kidney; the consequence of which necessarily was a greatly increased flow of blood to the remaining organ. An enumeration of the advantages afforded by the kidney for the prosecution of this inquiry would be very incomplete without some notice of the beautiful contrivance by means of which aqueous effusion naturally takes place into the uriniferous ducts; for an account of which we are indebted to my esteemed friend Mr. Bowman, of King's College. The piece of minute mechanism thus unexpectedly brought to light is in itself so exquisitely simple, and at the same time so admirably adapted to the accomplishment of the end it was intended to fulfil, that its discovery could not fail to elicit from every lover of natural science the warmest admiration.

But to myself this valuable addition to microscopical anatomy is fraught with a double interest. For it not only enables me to explain, and trace, the manner in which my experiments were productive of certain effects, but as a peculiar anatomical arrangement evidently connected with, and provided for, an important physiological purpose, it also constitutes a powerful argument in favour of the general hydraulic principles, which I have supposed to regulate many of the chief uses of the circulation. In the tuft of tortuous capillaries thus protruded into the extremity of each excretory tube, we have but an exaggeration, for a special object, of the general contrivance by which the lateral pressure of the blood contained in the terminating arterial ramifications is maintained at a point sufficient for the occurrence of effusion. It must be observed, that, in the healthy state, the lateral pressure induced by the impediments to the blood's passage through the convoluted vessels merely causes the constant exudation of its more aqueous portion into the surrounding tube. And by reflecting on this arrangement of the blood-vessels, and the natural absence of albuminous matters in the urine, the reader will find no difficulty in understanding the facts and reasoning which tend to demonstrate the connection between an increase in the lateral pressure of the blood contained in those vessels, and an effusion into the urinary passages of its various albuminous constituents in a ratio corresponding to that increased pressure.

Part V.

OF THE LAWS REGULATING EFFUSION.

It has been objected to some of the conclusions which were drawn from my experiments on venous obstruction, that the kidney operated on was necessarily exposed to an amount of disturbance which might possibly excite inflammation of the organ, and, in that case, the phenomena in question should be ascribed to the existence of that disease rather than to the mere physical disorder of the circulation. The very brief period which intervened between the performance of the experiment and the examination of the urine (being in many instances only a few minutes) might perhaps have furnished a sufficient answer to this supposition. But I thought it better to try the question fairly by a direct appeal to nature, and accordingly performed the two following experiments on rabbits of the average strength and condition.

Exp. 1. — The left kidney of a healthy rabbit was exposed in the usual manner, drawn out of the abdomen through the wound in the loins, cleared of the investing cellular tissue, and immediately afterwards returned; the wound being then closed by suture. The animal was killed at the end of an hour and a half. On being weighed, this kidney was found to be only nine grains heavier than the right; the weight of the latter being 73 grains, that of the former 82 grains. The left ureter presented nothing extraordinary in its appearance, being neither distended nor discoloured. The bladder contained six drachms of urine, which remained quite clear after the application of nitric acid and heat.

Exp. 2.—A precisely similar operation was performed on a rabbit of the same size, and the animal killed at the end of two hours and a half. The right kidney weighed 80 grains; and the left, the one exposed and handled, 84 grains; being an increase of only four grains. The bladder contained five drachms of opaque urine, which became quite clear on the addition of nitric acid.

The first law which I shall seek to establish on experimental evidence is the following; viz. That an obstruction to the return of blood through the renal vein will cause the presence of either liquid albumen, coagulating lymph, or blood in the urine secreted by a kidney otherwise healthy.

For this purpose I subjoin, in a tabular form, the results obtained in a number of experiments; a detailed account of all of which, with the exception of the two last, is contained in the 26th volume of the Medico-Chirurgical Transactions.

TABLE I.—*Exhibiting the Results of Twenty-one Experiments in which the Renal Vein was more or less completely obstructed.*

No. of experiment.	Interval between its performance and the examination of the urine.	Condition of the urine secreted by the affected kidney, so far as regards the presence in it of albumen, lymph, or blood.
1	10 minutes	Slightly albuminous.
2	30 minutes	Slightly albuminous.
3	30 minutes	No urine in bladder: ureter not examined.
4	10 minutes	Highly albuminous.
5	6 minutes	Very highly albuminous, and some slight appearance of lymph in the pelvis of the kidney.
6	3½ minutes	Bloody (taken from the ureter).
7	1 hour	Bloody.
8	1 hour	Slightly albuminous.
9	30 minutes	Highly albuminous.
10	7 minutes	Slightly albuminous.
11	1 hour	A mass of pellucid lymph in the bladder.
12	1 hour	Bloody, and contained a fibrinous coagulum.
13	1 hour	Water contained lymph and blood.
14	40 minutes	Bloody.
15	4½ days	Muddy, and faintly albuminous.
16	18 hours	Bloody.
17	1 hour	Bloody.
18	24 hours	Moderately albuminous.
19	2½ days	Reddened by blood, and highly albuminous.
20	2½ hours	Ureter contained a fibrinous coagulum, stained of a reddish colour at one point, and above it some highly albuminous urine.
21	2¼ hours	Bladder contained highly albuminous urine, which was also viscid and glairy; the ureter contained some distinctly fibrinous matter, which was perfectly transparent; one piece in size and appearance exactly resembled a particle of sago.

Now it will subsequently be shown that the results thus obtained precisely correspond with the phenomena generally admitted to constitute the primary effects of inflammation. Even coagulating lymph, the effusion of which is to this day mentioned by writers as the essential characteristic of that state, and as furnishing the only satisfactory distinction between it and congestion, will be seen to have occasionally followed the application of an impediment to the blood's passage through the smaller vessels of the kidney. The peculiar circumstance, which determines the production of one or other of the different effects met with, will soon be made apparent. But I may remark, that these experiments are, so far as my knowledge extends, the first in which the interesting, and—both in a therapeutical and pathological point of view—important process of the effusion of coagulating lymph has been traced to the operation of a purely physical cause.

In pursuance of the inquiry, I shall now proceed to show that the variety in the effects produced is not altogether dependent upon, nor explicable by, a difference in the degree of completeness of the obstruction. To be satisfied of this, it is only necessary to examine the following Table; which proves that the same degree of obstruction may, in different cases, be productive of very different effects.

TABLE II.—*Giving the Results of Eight Experiments, in all of which the Closure of the Renal Vein by Ligature was immediate and complete.*

No of experiment.	Marked in the previous table, No.	Interval between application of ligature and examination of the urine.	Condition of urine as regards the presence in it of albumen, lymph, or blood.
1	1	10 minutes	Slightly albuminous.
2	2	30 minutes	Do. Do.
3	4	10 minutes	Highly albuminous.
4	5	6 minutes	Very highly albuminous, and some appearance of lymph in the pelvis of the kidney.
5	6	$3\frac{1}{2}$ minutes	Bloody (taken from the ureter).
6	7	1 hour	Bloody.
7	20	$2\frac{1}{2}$ hours	Highly albuminous, and a fibrinous coagulum in the ureter.
8	21	$2\frac{1}{4}$ hours	Very highly albuminous; transparent fibrine in the ureter.

The facts contained in the first table having established the general principle, that an obstruction to the blood's return from the kidney will cause the presence, in the secretion of that organ, of one or more of certain substances evidently derived from the minute blood-vessels of the gland, the point which next presents itself for examination may be thus expressed, viz.:—To what, if any, physical cause are we to ascribe the different results met with in a number of experiments performed in precisely the same manner, and, so far as external circumstances are concerned, under the same conditions? We have, by the results presented in the last table, gained one negative answer to this question. And I now proceed to narrow the inquiry still further, by placing before the reader another table, which will prove that the nature of the effused products bears no proportion to the increase in the quantity of blood contained within the vessels of the organ, nor consequently to the amount of distension of those vessels.

TABLE III.—*Showing the relative Weights of the healthy and engorged Kidneys, with the Nature of the Changes observed in the Composition of the Secretion of the latter.*

No. of experiment; same as in first table.	Weight of healthy kidney in grains.	Weight of engorged kidney in grains.	Relative Weights	Condition of urine.
1	20	40	1—2	Slightly albuminous.
2	26	51	1—2 (?)	Do Do.
3	26	50		Not examined.
4	25	70	1—2	Highly albuminous.
5	25	50	1—2	Very highly albuminous, with lymph.
6	60	90	1—1·50	Bloody.
7	98	175	1—1·78	Bloody.
8	40	84	1—2·10	Slightly albuminous.
9	50	150	1—3	Highly albuminous.
10	42	73	1—1·73	Slightly albuminous.
11	100	130	1—1·30	A mass of clear lymph.
12	56	90	1—1·80	Bloody, with a fibrinous coagulum.
13	Not	ascertained.		
14	36	68	1—1·94	Bloody.
15	Not	ascertained.		
16	64	182	1—2·84	Bloody.
17	90	170	1—1·88	Bloody.
18 } 19 }	Not	ascertained.		
20	39	76	1—2 (?)	Highly albuminous, with fibrine.
21	46	92	1—2	Do. Do.

(When the urine is described as simply albuminous, it is to be inferred that there was no discolouration from any admixture of blood. Before weighing the kidneys, the vessels were divided close to their entrance into the organ, and the blood permitted to ooze from them; but no pressure was applied. The left kidney was, with one or two exceptions, that operated on; but I satisfied myself, by frequent comparisons, that there is no natural inequality between the weight of the two organs.)

From this last table, then, we may confidently infer that there is no relation between the nature of the effused matters, and the extent of the dilatation of the coats of the vessels, as measured by the quantity of blood they contain. And here I cannot avoid directing attention to the close resemblance which some of the results observed in these experiments bear to the phenomena noticed in chronic inflammation affecting the human subject. For in the latter case we also generally find the same inequality between the amount of local hyperæmia and the degree of intensity of the inflammatory attack, as indicated by its symptoms and immediate effects.

It having thus been shown that neither the degree of completeness of the obstruction, nor the extent of dilatation of the vessels, constitutes the peculiar cause of the difference in the results induced, let us now proceed to examine the only remaining physical agency to which that difference can possibly be ascribed. And, as calculated to elucidate the nature, operation, and source of this agency, it may be well briefly to consider the general effects produced by the obstruction of any freely-moving mass of fluid.

I have, throughout these investigations, had constant occasion to dwell upon and apply this general hydraulic principle; viz., that the degree of lateral pressure which a fluid exercises while traversing a tube, or system of tubes, is altogether dependent upon the relative facilities afforded for the influx and efflux of that fluid. And, as a corollary from this law, that any circumstance which tends to lessen the rate of discharge, while the rate of influx continues unaltered, will instantly, and in a very rapid ratio, increase the lateral pressure of the column of fluid till it becomes equal to the whole impelling force.

Now in the case of the fluid traversing the vessels of the living body, that impelling force is clearly derived from, and proportionate to the amount of, pressure of the general mass of aortic blood; which pressure is known to fluctuate very considerably, and sometimes very suddenly, from various circumstances, particularly those affecting the vigour and frequency of the heart's action. It follows, therefore, that the actual amount of lateral pressure with which each minute column of detained blood acts against the walls of its containing vessel, will, in every case of obstructed capillary circulation, be wholly regulated by two essential circumstances; viz., the degree of completeness of the local obstruction on the one hand, and the actual amount of impelling pressure then resident in the mass of arterial blood, on the other. The latter is, in all cases, evidently the *active* cause of a morbidly increased lateral pressure of the capillary blood-columns. But this tendency to an equal diffusion of the blood's pressure in the minute vessels, which is equivalent to either a total perversion or suspension of the healthy uses of the streams traversing them, is only observed when, from some cause disturbing the natural proportion between the rates of influx and efflux of the blood circulating through the vessels of the part, the rate of discharge of that fluid through the veins is not equal to its rate of influx through the arteries. Such a disproportion necessarily existed in all my experiments on the kidney; and the amount of lateral pressure of the columns of blood detained in the minute vessels of each, after the partial or complete closure of the vein, was—as in every other case of obstructed circulation—regulated thus. Assuming the impulse of the arterial blood to have been equal in a number of animals at the moment of performing the experiment, any difference in the amount of lateral pressure of the impeded columns of blood must then have been altogether dependent upon some inequality in the degree of obstruction existing in the renal vein of each. And on the other hand, where (as in the experiments comprised in Table II.) the obstruction was in several cases equally complete, the amount of lateral pressure of the stagnant masses of fluid was then necessarily quite equal to the onward pressure of each capillary blood-column, and, like it, wholly proportioned to the general pressure of the great mass of arterial blood.

But in examining how far this difference in the

lateral pressure of the blood contained in the vessels of the kidneys operated on is capable of explaining the variety in the effects produced, it is necessary to bear in mind the peculiar physical composition of that fluid while circulating in the vessels of a living animal. For general purposes it is sufficient to consider it as consisting of liquor sanguinis and red globules; but, in connection with the present inquiry, we must scrutinise more closely the composition of the former substance. It is this which gives to the blood all its peculiarities as a fluid; and in it also resides that self-coagulating power which distinguishes the vital from every other albuminous solution.

Now the liquor sanguinis, while in its natural state of motion, is, by a very simple process of physical analysis, clearly resolvable into three distinct portions, the constituent particles of which possess very different degrees of cohesive force. We have, first, a serosity or aqueous fluid, holding in solution various saline and animal matters, but no albumen. And, from the great mobility of its particles, this fluid is enabled to permeate with the greatest facility any porous structure; and is, in fact, naturally filtered through the coats of the Malpighian vessels in the form of urine.

The next ingredient of the liquor sanguinis is intermediate in its consistency between the aqueous fluid just described, and the still more cohesive self-coagulating albumen or fibrine. It corresponds to the serum of coagulated blood, and is identical with the coagulable lymph of old writers; being neither more nor less than a solution of albumen, and possessing, in common with all such solutions, much more viscidity than any simply aqueous liquid. Lastly, we have to notice the highly cohesive, self-solidifying substance which gives to the healthy blood its characteristic property of spontaneous coagulation. And so great is the tendency of the particles of this coagulating lymph to aggregate in masses, that the unceasing motion of the blood, in addition to its other important uses in the animal economy, is found to be essential to the preservation of the fluidity of the circulating mass.

From this variety in the cohesiveness of these three constituents of the liquor sanguinis, it is very evident that different degrees of force will be required for the expulsion of each through the same porous membrane. And even were there no collateral facts to support the conclusion, I do think that a common-sense view of the subject should impress every unprejudiced mind with the conviction that the effusion of one or other of these substances through the invisibly minute pores of the capillary membrane is, in every case, mainly regulated by the amount of lateral pressure, or expelling force, existing in the columns of fluid blood contained within those vessels.

The grounds on which this conclusion rests may be thus stated —:

1st. The impossibility of adducing any other rational physical explanation of the variety in the results met with, both in my experiments, and in cases of locally obstructed circulation in man and other animals. We must, therefore, in the absence of any other principle, either consent to adopt this law, or be satisfied to continue in a state of ignorance which is not the less complete from its being disguised beneath a mass of pompous but unmeaning words. This, it must be confessed, is only a negative argument in support of the proposition; but—

2ndly. It is an indisputable fact that in all obstructed blood-vessels there exists, behind the impediment, a mass of detained blood, the lateral pressure of which is unnaturally great. The immediate cause, therefore, to which I have assigned effusion is demonstrably true, so far as regards the fact of its existence, as an adequate expelling force, at that particular portion of the blood-vessels whence the exuded or extravasated matters are manifestly derived.

And, 3rdly, as it can be shown that the general force of the blood, both in different individuals and in the same individual at different times, is liable to very great changes in its amount, so also will the lateral pressure of the blood contained in any obstructed vessel be necessarily subjected to an equal range of variation. This fluctuation in the amount of lateral pressure of the minute blood-columns in different individuals will therefore explain the variety in the substances (constituents of the liquor sanguinis) expelled, through the porous membrane of the capillary vessels, in a number of cases of obstructed circulation. We may, consequently (reserving for future consideration some modifying circumstances), claim for the above-mentioned law a firmer foundation than mere negative evidence, and assert that, as it is possible to assign the varied phenomena in question to a cause demonstrably true and adequate to their production, it would be unphilosophical and useless to seek for any other till either the existence of that cause is disproved, or its operation is shown to be incompatible with the peculiar conditions of the case.

Part VI.

OF THE APPLICABILITY OF THE SAME LAWS TO THE EXPLANATION OF THE PHENOMENA, AND ELUCIDATION OF THE NATURE, OF INFLAMMATION.

Having thus, by a process of reasoning founded upon the ascertained laws of matter, and confirmed by numerous experiments upon the living body, established the general proposition, that a morbidly increased lateral pressure of the blood contained within the minute vessels of a part will, in a direct ratio to the amount of that increase, cause the exudation of either liquid albumen, or coagulating lymph, or the extravasation of blood, I now proceed to inquire how far the existence of the same physical disorder of the blood contained within the capillary vessels of an inflamed part may be considered to constitute the essential characteristic of that disease. But before attempting to ascertain, by a general examination of the subject, the compatibility of such a view with the known phenomena or attendant circumstances of the disease, it is of course indispensable that the fact of the existence, in every case of inflammation, of this local disorder in the distribution of the blood's pressure, should be clearly demonstrated.

Now whatever objections may be urged against the doctrine which recognises, in the local increase of the blood's lateral pressure, the essence of the disease termed inflammation, no one can deny the fact of the existence of an unnatural amount of distending or lateral pressure in the columns of blood filling the minute vessels of an inflamed part. For that there exists, in every case of inflammation, a certain amount of obstruction to the blood's passage through those vessels, is a conclusion which the united testimony of pathologists, and of microscopical observers, renders indisputable. And, the existence of that obstruction being once admitted, it follows as an inevitable consequence, that the lateral pressure of the fluid detained behind each impediment will be instantly increased in accordance with the physical laws so recently applied to the illustration of my experiments on the kidney.

It therefore only remains for me to examine how far the locally disordered physical condition of the blood thus shown to be a constant and necessary concomitant of inflammation, is referrible to the causes, productive of the symptoms and effects, and removable by the remedies found advantageous in the treatment, of that disease. And if I succeed in showing that this physical disorder of the blood corresponds in all these essential characteristics with the pathological condition ordinarily understood by the term inflammation, it must then remain for others to adduce reasons why that morbidly increased lateral pressure of the blood detained in the affected part should not be considered as identical with, and in itself the essence of, the disease so long designated by that ill-chosen word.

It has just now been remarked, that the existence of an obstruction to the blood's passage through the vessels of an inflamed part necessarily implies a morbid increase in the lateral pressure of the fluid columns thus detained. And as all modern pathologists more or less explicitly recognise the tendency of the causes of inflammation to induce, directly or indirectly, such an obstruction, I am, by this admission, spared the necessity of advancing any lengthened arguments in order to show that the action of those causes on the circulation of the part is such as to be inevitably followed by the peculiar physical disorder of the blood which I presume to constitute the essence of inflammation. So far, then, as my general proposition is concerned, any minute discussion of this point would be useless; but as a too exclusive attention to microscopical phenomena seems to me to have placed the mode of action of the exciting causes of this disease in an unnecessary amount of obscurity, a few remarks, having for their object the assignment of a fair and proper value to these observations, may not be altogether useless.

It must, then, in the first place, be remembered, that the disordered circulation observed in these experiments was almost invariably caused by the local application of some irritating substance. Any conclusions drawn from the unnatural phenomena then witnessed are, therefore, in strict reasoning, to be considered as illustrative of the action of only one class of the exciting causes of inflammation, viz. local sources of irritation.

Moreover the parts selected for observation are, from the very transparency which recommends them to the microscopist, evidently possessed of but a slight amount of vascularity, and consequently do not, in their diseased condition, exhibit such marked phenomena as would be presented by parts more copiously supplied with blood. And in most of the observations in question the irritant seems to have been applied to a very minute portion of the tissue under examination, apparently for the purpose of limiting its action to a small number of vessels.

Now, if we contrast these conditions with those existing in the generality of the cases of inflammation which we are called upon to treat in man, any inferences legitimately deducible from the observations in question must, I think, be considered as calculated to throw but a very faint light on the nature of those extensive and serious disorders of the circulation which, occurring in the highly vascular organs of the human body, produce such striking and injurious effects; for neither in their extent, intensity, nor causation, do the disorders thus artificially created correspond with the great majority of cases of inflammation presented to the medical practitioner.

There is, however, one microscopical phenomenon which cannot be passed over without a more detailed examination; I mean the appearance of an unnatural number of white globules in the blood contained within the affected vessels, together with a marked tendency in those globules to adhere to each other, and to the sides of the containing capillaries. This circumstance is, by many eminent writers, considered to indicate the possession by the blood present in an inflamed part of properties different from, or superadded to, its ordinary vital endowments, and which properties are presumed to be, in some inexplicable manner, connected with the production of the accompanying disease.

Now I am far from attempting to offer anything like an explanation of the nature and origin of these or any of the other minute particles which are described by microscopical pathologists under numerous names, as constituting the characteristic peculiarities of the various products of disease. In the present imperfect and confused state of our knowledge it is clearly impossible even to hazard an opinion as to the causes determining the production of each variety in the form, size, colour, and structure of the different microscopical bodies in question. For the discovery of any general laws explanatory of the appearance in one case of inflammation of certain peculiarly-formed globules or corpuscles, and their total absence in other cases under precisely similar perceptible conditions, we must have recourse to other sources of information in addition to microscopical observations. Analytical chemistry must lend its aid, by tracing (as far as its limited power will permit) the degree of connection existing between the appearance of each minute element of morbid development and the composition of the plasma and blood from which it is formed. And even where chemistry and the microscope fail to elucidate the point selected for examination, experiments on the living body—having the conditions of each so judiciously varied from those preceding it, and at the same time so skilfully combined, as invariably to lead to some definite conclusion—will, if I mistake not, be found to constitute a synthetical mode of investigation, by the aid of which results of striking novelty and vast importance may, in many instances, be rapidly attained. In short, the chemist, the microscopical observer, and the experimental pathologist, must co-operate in studying the nature of morbid actions; and it is only by the concentration of their respective energies upon the same point that we can ever hope to acquire any considerable number of sound pathological generalisations, or useful hygienic and therapeutical precepts.

But, to return from this slight digression to the consideration of the phenomenon which suggested these remarks; it does not, I think, involve any great deviation from the rules of correct reasoning to suppose that the power which, in the liquor sanguinis present in the vessels of an inflamed part evolves a mass of coherent globules, is, in its essential nature, not very far removed from that which induces the natural coagulation of the fibrinous portion of the blood. It can be shown that a local disorder of the blood's motion similar to that present in the incipient stage of inflammation (as described by microscopical observers) is, in other parts of the circulating system, productive of the same changes in the physical composition of that fluid as those now under consideration; for we know that in general the only condition required for the production of a fibrinous coagulum within any blood-vessel is a gradual and continued retardation of the stream of blood. In the large concretions formed in the heart and large vessels during a lingering death we have one instance of the operation of this law. But the successive fibrinous layers deposited on the internal surface of an aneurisimal sac exhibit a still closer resemblance to the phenomena presented in an inflamed part, inasmuch as the globules there manifest the same tendency to adhere to the walls of the containing vessel. This adhesion of the globules to the vascular walls seems to me to be mainly referable to the well-known fact, that the rate of motion of the external portion of a stream traversing any tube is always less than that of the central column: but it is by no means improbable that, from their similarity in chemical composition to the contiguous tissues, the so-called lymph globules may naturally possess a strong tendency to adhere to them under certain favourable conditions.

Now, all observers agree that the flow of blood through the vessels of an inflamed part is considerably slower than natural; we have, therefore, in this case also, that local retardation of the stream of blood which is recognised as capable of inducing the development and aggregation of fibrinous globules in other parts of the circulating system. And unless the opponents of this simple view of the subject are prepared to prove that the phenomena in question occur prior to, and quite independent of, that retardation of the blood's current, I cannot help thinking that it may be quite as philosophical to refer their production to a well-ascertained and familiar law, as to introduce on this particular occasion the mysterious and unintelligible operation of some new and indemonstrable agency. It may also be observed, that as the blood distributed in exceedingly minute columns throughout the capillaries is necessarily brought into contact with a much greater extent of vascular surface than that contained in the larger vessels, any natural attraction existing between that surface and the globules in question will, under similar circumstances, evidently operate most actively in the former portion of the circulating system.

In the next section of this paper I shall endeavour to show how determination of blood becomes a cause of inflammation; and the experiments already adduced prove that the existence of any great amount of venous obstruction will also give rise to the effects of the latter morbid state. It follows, therefore, that the exciting causes of inflammation may act by affecting the circulation through the larger vessels, arteries, or veins of the part, as well as by their direct influence on the capillaries; though it is only by the accumulation of a quantity of compressed blood in the latter thin porous vessels that the disease in question can be essentially constituted.

It will not require many words to exhibit the connection between the production of the symptoms of inflammation, and the existence of the local disorder of the circulation which I suppose to be identical with that disease.

The redness and swelling of the inflamed part are evidently direct effects of the distending force resulting from the increased lateral pressure of the detained columns of blood. The local pain and heat, being chiefly occasioned by an increased supply of arterial blood, are most marked in acute inflammation—the pathology of which will be more fully considered when reviewing the effects of determination of blood. But it may be observed, as a general rule, that the presence of these two symptoms in any case, and the degree of intensity in each, are mainly affected by a simple circumstance, viz. the preponderance of arterial or venous blood in the minute vessels of the part.

In continuation of this inquiry, we have, in the next place to examine the very interesting question, as to how far the immediate effects of inflammation are referrible to the peculiar physical condition of the blood contained in the minute vessels of the affected part. These effects are, by all modern pathologists, described as consisting in:—1. The exudation of a serous or aqueo-albuminous fluid. 2. The effusion of coagulating lymph. 3. The extravasation of blood. Now, the consideration of each of these phenomena at the length which its importance merits, is, on the present occasion, clearly impossible, inasmuch as it would involve the study of numerous difficult and complicated points connected with the pathology of dropsy, hæmorrhage, and the host of diseases originating in the exudation of coagulating lymph. I must, therefore, restrict myself to an attempt at demonstrating the dependence of these effects on the co-existing disorder of the circulation. The first point to be established is, the identity of the primary effects of inflammation, with those resulting from an unnaturally increased lateral pressure of the blood contained in the minute vessels of a part. And for this purpose it is only necessary to compare the phenomena just mentioned as constituting the immediate effects of the morbid condition designated by that word, with the results obtained in my experiments on the kidney, as described in the various tables. It must, in the next place, be shown that a tendency to a morbid increase in the lateral pressure of the blood contained in the affected part exists in every case of inflammation. And this tendency to an unnatural distribution of the blood's pressure in the capillaries, I have, in a preceding passage of this section, proved to be a necessary and inevitable consequence of that obstruction to the flow of blood through those vessels, which is universally recognised as an invariable accompaniment of the disease. This is, in fact, a self-evident proposition, if the existence of the local obstruction be admitted. It must therefore follow that the primary effects of inflammation, being identical with those produced by the unnatural condition of the blood so often alluded to, and which is, in some degree, always present in that disease, are clearly referrible to that co-existing physical cause. Some remarks on the connection between the amount of increase in the lateral pressure of the capillary blood-columns, and the production of each effect, will interfere less with the general argument if deferred for a short time.

It now only remains to consider how far the remedies found useful in the treatment of inflammation are calculated to remove that local disorder of the circulation which invariably accompanies, and which I suppose to be identical with, that disease. The general principles of the treatment will be more fully discussed hereafter; but it is impossible to avoid noticing how closely the measures sanctioned by the experience of ages accord with the therapeutic indications which spring directly from the pathological views now advanced, as to the nature of inflammation. For, with the exception of mercury and a few other articles of the materia medica, of whose mode of operation we are wholly ignorant, the remedies employed with success in the treatment of inflammation, will all be found to act by restoring the natural balance of the pressures acting on either surface of the capillary blood-vessels. Now the most important pathological phenomenon which results from the existence of this disease, and the prevention and removal of which constitutes the chief object of our treatment, is the effusion into the adjacent cellular tissue of the serous and fibrinous portions of the blood. This effusion I have before stated to arise—1st, directly, from an increased lateral pressure of the blood contained within the minute porous vessels of the part; and 2ndly, indirectly, by diminished support to, or pressure on, the exterior of those vessels. It is evident, therefore, that a successful plan of treatment must embrace, and be based upon an observance of the two opposite conditions to those just specified. We accordingly, as the general principles of treatment endeavour — 1st, to diminish the lateral pressure of the blood contained in the minute vessels of the inflamed part; 2ndly, to increase the pressure acting on the exterior of those vessels.

The first point is attained by blood-letting, purgatives, and all other evacuants; by digitalis, colchicum, and other substances which possess the power of reducing the heart's action; and, after depletion in strong subjects, or primarily in asthenic systems, by derivatives or counter-irritants. These measures, with the exception of the last-mentioned group, act by diminishing the general pressure of the arterial blood in the system; derivatives can of course only indirectly reduce the pressure of the blood-columns in the inflamed part by diverting a larger proportion of the arterial blood to other vessels.

The measures which accomplish the second indication are, mechanical support, friction, cold, and astringents. The removal of any sources of impediment to the return of blood from the part, and an attention, where practicable, to its position, are beneficial observances, which are of course in perfect unison with the preceding therapeutic principles.

The result of this examination is, I think, the perfect demonstration of the truth of my proposition —that the morbidly increased lateral pressure of the capillary blood-columns, which invariably accompanies inflammation, is directly referrible to the causes, productive of the symptoms and effects, and relieved by the measures adopted for the treatment of that disease. What then, I ask, constitutes the distinction between the group of pathological phenomena designated by the word inflammation, and the local disorder in the physical condition of the blood which occasions those symptoms and effects? Or, which more correctly represents the disease? For, in the one case, we have described a deviation from the natural state of the local circulation, which can be shown to constitute the connecting link between the operation of the causes, and the production of the effects of a certain pathological condition: while, in the other, we are told to recognise, in certain visible effects of an imperceptible and unknown cause, a disease the essential nature, seat and origin of which are buried in obscurity. I contend therefore, that the peculiar physical disorder of the blood contained in the minute vessels of the affected part, constitutes that central link in the chain of causes and effects which was required to complete our knowledge of the pathology of inflammation. And by the recognition of this as the morbid condition essentially constituting that disease, much of the darkness now enveloping the causation of numerous pathological phenomena will be dispelled, many conflicting opinions and modes of treatment will be reconciled, and a new lustre will be reflected on that glorious discovery, without which, these disorders must ever have remained vital and unintelligible mysteries.

So far, then, as relates to the study of the nature of inflammation, any further remarks on the present occasion would perhaps be unnecessary; but it is impossible to leave this subject without alluding to congestion, a local disorder of the circulation, admitted to bear a close resemblance to, but at the same time considered essentially distinct from, inflammation. In the literal acceptation of the word, congestion is evidently synonymous with hyperæmia; and, as this latter state also exists in inflammation, pathologists seem to have been not a little puzzled to lay down any clear and satisfactory method of distinguishing the two affections. And it will not, I think, be found a very difficult task to show that these two disorders of the capillary circulation are different forms of the same pathological condition; the distinction between them being founded on the degree of intensity, and not on any material variety in the nature, of the abnormal state constituting the disease.

For the sole characteristic phenomenon now relied upon by pathologists, as affording the means of distinguishing between inflammation and congestion, is the absence of fibrinous exudation in the latter morbid state, while it is represented as being an invariable accompaniment of the former. And in proof of the accuracy of this representation of the prevalent opinion on the question, it is only necessary for me to refer to the writings of Alison, Travers, Bennett, and others. Now, in my experiments on the kidney, I have met with fibrinous coagula in the urinary passages, and in one instance with a considerable quantity of coagulating lymph, as the effects of what I have been content to term an unnatural increase in the lateral pressure of the columns of blood contained within the minute vessels of that gland. I have, at the risk of appearing unnecessarily tedious, repeatedly alluded to this as the immediate cause of every species of effusion; others seem to prefer terming it a state of congestion. But, however we may designate the pathological state, the fact of fibrinous exudation occurring as one of its effects destroys the value of that phenomenon as peculiarly distinctive of inflammation. As will be seen from the experiments mentioned in the following part of this communication, the same pathological phenomena have followed the congestion of the renal vessels, whether that increased lateral pressure of the capillary blood-columns arose from venous obstruction, or from an artificially augmented flow of blood through the renal artery. It is true that the quantity of fibrine thus obtained was in many instances very minute, and that in several experiments it did not appear at all. But this circumstance is fully explicable by the difficulty of maintaining, at will, the pressure of the blood at the required point, and no higher, for a sufficient length of time. And one positive fact must, in experiments on a question of this kind, be considered to counterbalance a thousand failures. I contend, therefore, that this distinction between congestion and inflammation can no longer be maintained; for that whenever an adequate amount of compressing or expelling force acts upon the blood contained in the minute vessels of any part, the exudation of the fibrinous portion of the liquor sanguinis will then invariably take place. It is a purely mechanical process, and, as such, regulated by physical laws. We must, then, in order to explain its occurrence in some cases of obstructed capillary circulation, and its absence in others, trace the operation of the various physical and vital laws affecting the pressure of the blood contained within the minute vessels of the part, and not remain content with ascribing the variety in the effects witnessed to unknown and undemonstrable differences in the nature of the two disorders.

I might have added Dr. Billing's name to those of the other pathologists who suppose congestion to be distinguished from inflammation by the presence of fibrinous effusion in the latter, and its absence in the former case. But he is evidently disposed to attach less importance than the generality of writers on inflammation, to the maintenance of a distinction between the two disorders. For he speaks of them as "but varieties of distended vessels," and admits "the impossibility of drawing a line between inflammation and congestion, the one passing into the other by insensible shades."

And Dr. C. J. B. Williams, in his last work ("Principles of Medicine"), when speaking of the effects of congestion as existing in the kidney and elsewhere, advances views precisely identical with those which I had been led to entertain, both from the results of my experiments and from a general review of the circumstances connected with the pathology of granular disease of that organ. Thus, after remarking that the cause producing effusion is "distension of the vessels," and alluding to the influence of the "condition" or composition of the blood in modifying the nature of the effused matters, he proceeds to observe*, — "The same circumstances determine the character of the effused fluid. Where the blood is poor, the watery parts easily pass from congested vessels even without much distension, and contain but little albumen. But if the blood abounds in the protein compounds, more pressure is required before much effusion takes place; and then, when the pressure is great, the fluid effused often contains not only albumen in large proportion, but self-coagulating fibrin also.†" . . . . . . "Fluxes arising from congestion of high tension exhibit an unusual amount of animal matter of an albuminous or mucous kind, as instanced in a bronchorrhœa, mucous diarrhœa, and leucorrhœa. I have been almost induced to suppose that the polypous concretions and pseudo-membranous films occasionally effused on mucous surfaces may result from long-continued congestion. I have seen these evacuated from the air-tubes in one case, and in another

* Principles of Medicine, pp. 148, 149. London, 1843.
† Ibid p. 138.

from the intestines, from time to time, for months, and even years, without symptoms of inflammation, but under circumstances rendering it probable that congestion was present.*" Nevertheless, while thus referring to congestion as to an adequate cause, the phenomenon considered by all other pathologists as essentially characteristic of inflammation, Dr. Williams still endeavours to establish a distinction between these two pathological states. And, as will be seen by a glance at the subjoined definitions, this distinction is founded upon a difference in the velocity or relative motion of the blood contained in the minute vessels of the part. Thus, congestion is defined as "excess of blood in a part, with diminished motion of that blood." Inflammation, as "too much blood in a part, with motion (of that blood) partly increased, partly diminished." Now, even by the author's own admission, the same state of the circulation, *in the vessels of the affected part*, exists in *both* disorders; for we have in each local hyperæmia, with a retardation or tendency to stagnation of that accumulated blood. The distinction is, therefore, wholly based upon the state of the circulation *in the adjacent vessels.*

And, in fact, this definition of inflammation seems to me to be merely a description of the immediate effects on the local circulation of the obstruction of a few vessels, at a moment when the heart's action is tolerably vigorous. The phenomena described are therefore precisely what might have been expected

* Principles of Medicine, p. 169. London, 1843.

to be visible under the microscope, when a minute quantity of some irritating substance is applied to the transparent structures of any animal. In this case, however, as the obstruction is produced through the action of an irritant on the vital properties of the contractile tissues, the resulting pathological state is termed *inflammation*. Whereas, if the same physical phenomena followed the application of any purely *mechanical* cause of obstruction, such as pressure, or the ligature of a vein, the morbid state produced would, I presume, then be considered an instance of mere *congestion*. But as the ultimate effect of both classes of causes is the same, the only difference being that in the one case the local disorder of the circulation is a direct and immediate, in the other an indirect and secondary, consequence of their application, I cannot acquiesce in Dr. Williams' views on this point, nor can I perceive, in the circumstances dwelt upon by him, any adequate ground for regarding inflammation and congestion as two distinct diseases. For that increased motion of the blood in the surrounding vessels is a purely physical phenomenon, explicable on common hydraulic principles, and resulting from the additional force imparted to those columns of blood by the constant rush or flow through the anastomosing channels of the fluid pent up and accumulated in the vessels leading to the obstructed capillaries.

It being thus, I think, rendered evident that inflammation and congestion are but two forms of the same disease, differing from each other in the *intensity*, and not in the *nature* of the pathological condition essentially constituting them, we must now assign some precise signification to the latter term, as it will probably still be used in medical writings. But before doing so, it is necessary to refer to an arrangement of cases of congestion sometimes observed by authors; I mean, their division into active and passive. Now the local disorder of the circulation, to which the term *active* congestion is applied, seems to me to be identical with that generally known as determination of blood, the pathology of which will be considered in the following part of this inquiry; while the term *passive* congestion I consider to express the existence of *a state of capillary hyperæmia, without much increase in the lateral pressure of that accumulated blood.* And when the term *chronic* is used to denote the *intensity*, and not the *duration* of inflammation, the pathological condition then present is very similar to that just described. I may here observe, that it is an error to suppose that the capillary congestion resulting from venous obstruction cannot produce the same morbid effects as that occasioned by any other cause; for the experiments so often referred to suffice to prove that the exudation of lymph is as clearly an effect of venous obstruction as the effusion of serum, or the extravasation of blood. Dr. Bennett, of Edinburgh, a recent and an able writer on inflammation, but who, like the great majority of pathologists and physiologists of the present day, trusts, perhaps, too exclusively to *unaided* *observation*, has the following remarks on this subject:—"Why it should happen that venous congestions are never accompanied by an exudation of blood-plasma, whilst arterial congestions are, is a point that no one has yet endeavoured to explain. To me it appears certain that all inflammatory effusions occur through the capillary or intermediate vessels, and not in such vessels as may be properly called arteries or veins. . . . . But it is scarcely possible to suppose that the mechanical difference in the density of the filtrating membrane should constitute the only distinction. It is impossible to reconcile the phenomena without having recourse to some active vital power of attraction between the blood and the parenchyma, as formerly explained; a power which, operating in the one case and not in the other, causes different constituents of the blood to become exuded. We are compelled, in all our considerations of the subject, to go back to this explanation as to an ultimate fact."* Now, with respect to the above-mentioned difference in the effects of arterial and venous congestions, instead of endeavouring to explain its occurrence, I must dispute the fact; for extreme and continued *venous* congestion must necessarily be followed by *capillary* congestion; and if the lateral pressure of the blood detained in these delicate porous vessels be sufficiently great, the effusion or exudation of coagulating lymph will most certainly take place. I have extracted the other

* A Treatise on Inflammation as a Process of Anormal Nutrition, p 39. Edinburgh, 1844.

sentences from Dr. Bennett's work, for two reasons. In the first place, they represent, in a concise and clear manner, the views entertained on this question by many eminent pathologists; and they at the same time afford an instance of that preference of a *vital* to a physical, a mysterious to a simple, explanation of a given phenomenon, which, manifested as it so generally is by the most distinguished and talented members of our profession, cannot but exercise a very injurious influence on the progress of medical science. Having been thus candid in pointing out what I conceive to be a defect in Dr. Bennett's pathological reasoning, I cannot avoid expressing an opinion that his short treatise on inflammation presents a more complete and intelligible view of the subject, and is, at the same time, characterised by closer reasoning and more careful discrimination, than any other work which has yet fallen under my notice.

The preceding remarks will, I hope, suffice to establish the principle that the production of one or other of the immediate effects of inflammation is, in every case, *mainly* determined by the amount of pressure acting on the columns of blood contained in the capillaries of the affected part. If, therefore, it were always in our power to ascertain during life the nature of the accompanying effusion, we should have a very simple and natural arrangement of cases of inflammation under three heads, denoting as many shades of difference in the intensity of the disease. Acute inflammation could then be defined as capillary hyperæmia, with more or less extensive extravasation of blood; sub-acute inflammation would be that form of the disease in which the effusion of liquor sanguinis was the preponderating morbid phenomenon; and atonic, or asthenic, either of which is a better term than chronic inflammation, being a state of mere congestion, would present only a serous or aqueo-albuminous effusion. In some instances it may be possible to recognise this natural classification even during life, and, when practicable, some advantage may be found from its observance, as calculated to suggest the remedies best suited to the particular form of the disease then under examination. But as, in the majority of cases of internal inflammation, we cannot avail ourselves of this means of diagnosis, our opinion as to the relative intensity of the attack must be necessarily drawn from a consideration of other circumstances. And even were it always possible to use this general rule, it would require to be very much modified in its application to particular cases, by a constant reference to the anatomical structure of the part affected, the composition of the blood, and integrity of structure of its coloured globules, and various other considerations.

I mentioned, towards the commencement of this paper, that Mr. J. W. Earle had promulgated some views on the nature of inflammation very similar to those which I had been led to adopt. The parts of his communication which bear the greatest resemblance to my conclusions, will be found at pages 107 and 108 of the 16th volume of the MEDICAL GAZETTE. But as he reasons upon the supposition that the capillaries have no proper coats, being mere channels or grooves in a contractile parenchyma, I cannot very clearly understand how the process of effusion is to be accomplished. In a subsequent passage of his paper (p. 141), Mr. Earle, in support of his very mechanical doctrine as to the formation of pus, endeavours to show that the several parts of the blood exude in the order of their fluidity; "the finest and most fluid first, and the coarsest last." But he certainly carries the idea too far when he represents the red globules as passing in their turn through the minute pores of the parenchyma, and becoming there converted into pus-globules by the mechanical detention of their colouring matter in the meshes of the sieve through which they have to pass.

It is scarcely necessary to add that the present inquiry embraces only the first stage of inflammation, in which the blood detained in the obstructed vessels retains more or less fluidity, and is consequently subjected to hydro-dynamic laws. With the coagulation of the blood in its vessels the process of effusion ceases; and the changes which the effused matters and the solidified blood subsequently undergo form a branch of pathological inquiry totally distinct from that which I proposed to undertake on the present occasion. But even from the little attention which it has been in my power to give to this subject, I feel convinced that an investigation of the pathology of the *secondary effects* of inflammation, conducted on the principles previously indicated, could not fail to afford most important and interesting results. At present, the object which seems chiefly to engage the attention of pathologists is the determination of the order in which these changes occur, and of the nature of the minute structural peculiarities accompanying each. But is it not possible, as it is most undoubtedly desirable, to attain that higher and more beneficial knowledge, by means of which we may be enabled to refer the production of each one of these morbid effects to its own peculiar determining causes, and thus, to a certain extent, perhaps ultimately acquire the power of regulating, in each case of unsubdued inflammation, the nature of its ultimate termination?

Having thus endeavoured to demonstrate the pathological condition which essentially constitutes inflammation, and to explain the production of its immediate effects, I shall reserve some remarks on the influence of these views upon its treatment until the subject of determination of blood has been fully examined. It will be seen that I consider the mechanism and forces operating in the production of the immediate effects of inflammation to be identical with those which I previously pointed out as causing nutritive effusion. The only difference between the healthy and the morbid process is in the extent of the effusing surface and the intensity of the expelling pressure; and, as the consequence of these changes, an increase in the quantity of blood-plasma exuded. Hence my views on this point are substantially identical with those of Dr. Bennett and the majority of pathologists. But the phenomena which they regard as the effect of an unknown vital power, I am content to refer to the operation of a very simple physical cause. With them, however, I consider inflammation to be, in its essence, merely "an extreme degree of a natural and healthy action . . . occurring in parts where, or under circumstances when, its continuance is likely to disturb the nervous system, and thus affect the health of the individual, or to prove injurious or inconvenient from the effects to which it may give rise."*

Part VII.

OF THE MORBID EFFECTS PRODUCED BY AN UNNATURALLY INCREASED PRESSURE OF THE BLOOD CONTAINED WITHIN THE ARTERIAL SYSTEM.

Having thus endeavoured to show that an anormal increase in the lateral pressure of the blood contained within the *minute* vessels of the affected part, is the immediate cause of those pathological phenomena which are considered to constitute the disease termed inflammation, it now remains to examine the operation of the causes which produce that allied local disorder of the circulation generally known as determination of blood.

This disorder, as its name implies, is an effect of

* An Inquiry, &c. p. 61.

an unequal distribution of the blood, and *consists in the accumulation of an unnatural quantity of that fluid in the arteries of a particular part*—the capillarics or minute porous vessels being comparatively unaffected. In their essential nature, and in the operation of their causes, determination and inflammation are very similar; the chief difference between them being constituted by the pathological phenomena which they respectively occasion. And this variety in their effects is a natural consequence of the different physical properties possessed by the affected vessels. For the thin membrane forming the parietes of the capillaries readily admits of the exudation of liquor sanguinis when in a state of unnatural compression, while the thickness and density of the proper arterial tunics effectually prevent the escape through them of any portion of the contained blood.

Before, however, considering the questions connected with determination of blood, it is necessary to refer to an analogous disorder of the circulation, of which the aorta itself is occasionally the seat. And the study of this physical peculiarity of the great mass of arterial blood is the more interesting, as it illustrates the operation of the causes producing a similar condition of the blood contained within the smaller vessels of the arterial system.

In a former paper on the physiology of the cirenlation, I pointed out the circumstances which influence the amount of lateral pressure exercised by the mass of blood contained in the aorta, and further observed, that " as this force is equally affected by a change in the condition of the heart, or of the smaller vessels, both which changes are continually occurring, it may, in the same individual, be at one time so slight as to be incapable of accomplishing its healthy uses, while at another period its distending power may be so considerable, as to rupture some of the containing vessels, and thus threaten the destruction of life."

The present communication having for its chief object the elucidation of the pathology of those forms of disordered circulation which consist essentially in a general or partial obstruction to the proper passage of the blood, we cannot here consider those cases in which, from a deficient accumulation of fluid in the aorta, the functions dependent on the distension of its elastic walls are imperfectly performed. But the omission of any further allusion to this point is the more excusable, as this disorder is perhaps more interesting, from its presenting an instance of the confirmation of a physiological law by pathological phenomena, than important as an agent operating in the production of structural disease.

From the principles previously established it follows, very evidently, that an increased lateral pressure of the blood contained in the aorta can only arise from one or other of two classes of causes —viz., either from causes which tend to induce a more rapid influx of blood by quickening the contractions of the ventricle, or from circumstances calculated to diminish the efflux of arterial blood by affecting the calibre, through the contractility, of the minute discharging tubes. And causes of each kind will, of course, occasionally co-operate in their action.

The causes accelerating the flow of blood into the aorta are, with the exception of bodily exercise and certain medicinal stimulants, chiefly of an emotional nature. That the force and frequency of the ventricular contractions are at once increased by anger and other passions, is a fact familiar to every one. And it must also be evident to every careful observer, that the lateral pressure of the aortic blood is at the same time augmented, and that this occurs in a ratio more or less intimately connected with the *abruptness of the application*, as well as with the intensity or power of the exciting cause of the quickened circulation. In no other manner can we explain the bursting of blood-vessels, so long noticed as an occasionally fatal effect of a fit of anger, or the equally striking instances recorded by surgical writers, in which ligatures upon large arteries have been displaced, and fatal hæmorrhage thus induced, in consequence of the patients being either affected by powerful mental emotion, yielding to the passions, or making some violent muscular effort. And, to take cases of more frequent occurrence, who has not during exercise personally experienced the very different sensations caused by a gradual and a sudden increase in the action of the heart? In the one case the arteries and capillaries seem readily to accommodate their calibre to the gradually increased quantity of blood poured into the aorta, and the only sensation induced by the accelerated circulation is a not unpleasant glow in the thorax, rapidly diffusing itself over the whole body. But when a person starts at once from a state of perfect repose to the performance of some feat requiring great and continued muscular exertion, various distressing and inconvenient phenomena immediately result. Under such circumstances the violent palpitation and tumultuous action of the heart, the painful distension felt in the cardiac region, and the unnatural pulsation of the large arteries, without any corresponding disorder of the circulation through the small arteries and capillaries, sufficiently evince the existence of a morbid accumulation of blood in the great arterial trunks. And the hurried panting respiration, and occasional expectoration of blood (if the person be at all plethoric), show that the pulmonary circulation is similarly affected. The difficulty which the blood thus experiences in passing from the aorta into the smaller arteries is evidently occasioned by the resisting contractility of the capillary vessels; but as the same cause operates in the production of determination of blood, it may be most advantageously considered when speaking of the analogous disorder of the circulation through the smaller arteries.

Of those causes of an increased lateral pressure of the aortic blood which act by diminishing the efflux from the arterial system, the sudden application of cold to the extremities and surface of the body is perhaps the most frequent. And the contraction of the innumerable cutaneous capillaries, which we witness as its immediate effect, by rendering those vessels incapable of transmitting the usual quantity of blood, must necessarily cause an accumulation of that fluid in the large arterial trunks. The experiments of Poiseuille, moreover, show that under such circumstances the heart exercises a compensating power, increasing the force of its contractions so much as to raise the pressure of the aortic blood considerably above its natural amount. In some instances, where the bent tube was applied to the carotid after ligature of the aorta, the mercury indicated a pressure double the amount of that which had been previously observed. And the effect of the temporary obliteration of a great number of minute vessels upon the condition of the aortic blood is precisely similar, though of course less intense in degree.

In whatever manner produced, this unnatural amount of pressure of the aortic blood, acting equally in every direction, may occasion morbid effects, from its distending influence upon the coats of the aorta; or it may affect the heart from its backward pressure; or it may cause the accumulation of an unnatural quantity of blood in the smaller arteries of the body. Each of these effects is worthy of a brief consideration, and the third is particularly interesting, from its presenting, on a more extended scale, those phenomena which, when confined to the arteries of a particular part or organ, constitute determination of blood.

The thick elastic walls of the aorta are, in their healthy state, so admirably adapted to the peculiar position of that vessel in the circulating apparatus, that their rupture under the distending pressure of the contained blood is never witnessed but as the result of arterial disease. It is true that we occasionally find great dilatation of the whole tube near its attachment to the heart, but it would appear almost a physical impossibility that any amount of lateral pressure which the arterial blood might derive from the ventricular impulse could, in the natural state of the aortic coats, induce their laceration. In cases, however, where their strength and elasticity have been diminished by previous disease, this force may and does occasion their rupture at the weakened points, and thus becomes the immediate cause of aneurism. And the same dilating pressure continuing to act upon the attenuated coats of the aneurismal sac, induces that laceration which generally conducts these cases to a fatal issue.

But, in addition to its well-known action as the immediate or proximate cause of aneurism, it is, I think, almost certain that an habitual increase in the pressure of the arterial blood exercises an important influence in predisposing to that disease. And statistical observations, by showing its more frequent occurrence in men than in women, and the peculiar liability to it of sailors and others whose occupation requires violent and sudden muscular exertion, contribute, with the fact of its most generally appearing during the prime of life, to give considerable support to the opinion. As a predisposing cause of aneurism this force may operate *directly*, by causing a certain amount of fibrinous exudation through the lining membrane of the aorta into the cellular space between it and the middle coat; or it may *indirectly* occasion the same effect, through the nutritious vessels or vasa vasorum. In either case the changes occurring in the patches of effused fibrine may be productive of the various physical and chemical alterations of structure which precede, and predispose to, the formation of an aneurismal pouch. A very slight consideration of the constant and reciprocal relation existing between the force and frequency of the ventricular contractions, and the amount of pressure of the aortic blood, will render it evident that any great increase in the latter force must inevitably produce considerable disorder of the heart's action. For the power exercised by the great instrument of the circulation in propelling the blood, varies with the resistance offered to the entrance of that blood into the aorta; and this resistance arises from the backward pressure of the fluid previously contained in that vessel. With the diminution of that pressure the contractions of the ventricle, in the absence of unnatural stimuli, become less frequent and less powerful; and the state of the circulation during sleep furnishes an interesting example of the operation of this law. But if, either from inordinate action of the heart itself, or from diminished calibre of the smaller vessels, the general and therefore the backward pressure of the aortic blood be unnaturally increased, the same compensating principle, continuing in operation, may give rise to very injurious and even fatal consequences. It has long been known that, in certain debilitated states of the system, a very slight exertion may cause momentary exhaustion and syncope; and where the constitution is very much enfeebled, as in mercurial erythismus, this syncope may be fatal. Now since a trifling increase in the resisting pressure of the aortic blood suffices, in these cases, to deprive the heart of its power of contraction, why may not the extraordinary obstruction to the flow of blood from the ventricle, constituted by the mass of fluid accumulated in the aorta during excessive and prolonged mental excitement or muscular exertion, occasion the same effect in an individual previously in the enjoyment of tolerable or even perfect health? And I cannot but think that, in many cases of sudden death, where no morbid appearances are perceptible, the fatal occurrence is referrible to a paralysis of the heart consequent on this physical disorder of the circulation. It is certainly the most frequent immediate cause of death in all forms of heart disease, when the life of the individual has for a long time been, as it were, supported by a single thread. And in all chronic diseases, where the powers of life are slowly exhausted, a trifling addition to the pressure of the aortic blood, by inducing the dissipation of the slight remnant of contractile power yet possessed by the heart, is often the action which ushers in the fatal catastrophe.

But, irrespective of its exhausting influence upon the contractile power of the heart, this physical disorder of the mass of arterial blood operates as the immediate cause of the most common forms of ventricular disease. For whether there be simple hypertrophy of the ventricle, or hypertrophy with dilatation, or enlargement of the ventricular cavity with attenuation of its parietes, the pathological condition is, in each case, distinctly referrible to the resistance or backward pressure of the aortic blood as its universal and proximate cause. And in the treatment of every form of heart disease, the prevention of a morbid accumulation of blood in the aorta, and the diminution of the pressure of the fluid mass to a point as low as is consistent with the proper performance of its physiological uses, constitute hygienic and therapeutic principles of the greatest importance.

We have now to consider the third effect of an unnatural increase in the pressure of the aortic blood; viz. an unusual accumulation of fluid in, and consequent distension of, the rest of the arterial system. While walking, or taking any other kind of moderate exercise, we can, by our sensations and by the greater pulsation of the superficial arteries, trace the gradual passage of the accumulated blood from the aorta into the smaller arterial branches. In these cases the accumulation consequent on the increased disproportion between the influx and efflux of arterial blood merely occasions a slight increase in the calibre of the smaller vessels, and a more rapid circulation through the capillaries and veins, with increased activity of the various functions served by the columns of blood traversing the former vessels. But when, as during violent exercise, the pressure of the arterial blood is more considerable, it not only induces inordinate pulsation of the different arteries, but also occasionally causes extravasation of blood from the rupture of some of the smaller and weaker vessels;

and, under these circumstances, it is also very apt to disorder the functions of the capillary blood-currents. Thus, after running for some time, if unused to the exercise, or at all plethoric, a small quantity of blood is not unfrequently expectorated even by young and healthy individuals. Fibrinous exudations, the effect of the same physical cause, are also often found in the serous cavities of animals which have been fattened for the market and driven some distance; and, from the following accidental observation, I conclude that an albuminous condition of the urine will frequently be found in animals hunted to death. Two young rabbits which had been kept in a large room with some older ones were found dead, and, from the superficial wounds present on their bodies, had evidently been destroyed by the stronger animals. In both instances the urine, which was tested from motives of curiosity, contained a considerable quantity of albumen, copious flakes appearing on the application of heat and nitric acid.

It is very evident that these morbid phenomena are the immediate and ordinary effects of an increased lateral pressure of the columns of blood contained within the smaller vessels; and it can also be readily understood that the same distending force which ruptures a small but impermeable artery, and thus causes the escape of the blood *en masse*, will, if less intense, and acting on a finer and more porous vessel, occasion the exudation either of liquor sanguinis, or of a simply albuminous fluid. But it is now necessary to consider the circumstance which prevents the compressed and accumulated blood from escaping freely into the veins, and thus maintains the unnatural amount of pressure of the arterial columns. When enumerating, in a former paper, the natural obstacles to the circulation, I mentioned the contractility of the smaller vessels as one of the most considerable, and represented it as a power opposed to, and constantly resisting, the action of the heart. The phenomena of a languishing circulation, which were first described by Spallanzani, are, I think, almost conclusive on this point; for, in these cases, the capillary blood-columns, during that slow and feeble action of the heart which precedes death, are seen to advance synchronously with each ventricular contraction, and to recede immediately afterwards, the alternate preponderance of the impelling and repelling forces giving the blood an oscillatory movement. It is true that the elasticity of the tissues may, to a certain extent, co-operate with their contractility in the production of this effect; but the influence of either property upon the passage of the blood through them must be the same. Each must necessarily oppose—it cannot assist—the circulation of the blood. The possession of contractility by the minute blood-vessels being, then, incontestable, it might naturally have been expected that they will also be subject to the physiological and pathological laws common to all other forms of contractile tissue. But, since the decline of Cullen's doctrine of a spasm of the extreme vessels as the proximate cause of fever and inflammation, there has been an evident disposition to regard the capillaries as differing materially in their vital endowments and susceptibilities from the other contractile structures of the body; and, though the vascular tunics, being subservient to functions different from those of the higher forms of contractile tissue, do undoubtedly exhibit a corresponding peculiarity in their action, it does appear to me that the pathological distinction which now separates these varieties of the same vital structure has been too hastily assumed, and has never been satisfactorily established by facts or reasoning. For the explanation of the phenomena now under consideration, it is not necessary to claim for the minute vessels a liability to actual spasm; it will suffice for my present purpose that they be allowed to possess, in common with every other contractile tube or cavity, the power or property of resisting any attempt at their *sudden* and forcible dilatation; and it must remain for those who are inclined to dispute this proposition to adduce their reasons for considering these vessels as exempt from the operation of a general and well-established law.* This principle, then, operating in the contractile capillaries, as in all

* Many surgical operations demonstrate the necessity of attending to the influence of *time* in modifying the action of dilating or extending forces upon contractile tissue. Thus, in the reduction of a dislocated limb, or in the injection of the bladder, or any other muscular cavity, it is found that while a slowly-applied elongating power acts without experiencing any resistance from the contractility of the yielding tissues, the abrupt application of a similar force becomes, in fact, *a mechanical stimulus*, and, as such, instantly causes an extreme contraction of the muscular structures. It is from the operation of a similar exciting cause that the capillaries, under the circumstances above mentioned, resist the influx of the arteria

similar structures of the body, enables us to understand how a *suddenly* increased influx of blood, consequent on an excited action of the heart, causes a morbid accumulation of fluid in, and distension of, the arterial system, while an almost equal increase in the activity of the circulation, *if slowly and gradually induced*, may exist without the production of any unpleasant or injurious consequences.

Passing from the study of the pathological phenomena following an unnatural accumulation of blood in the aorta and general arterial system, we have now to examine some of the questions connected with a similar derangement of the circulation in the arteries of a particular part or organ. That an undue accumulation of blood in these vessels, with increased pressure of the detained fluid, and, consequently, increased rapidity of the capillary blood-currents, is the pathological condition essentially constituting the local disorder known as determination of blood, cannot, I think, be doubted; for the unusual fulness of the arteries of the part is, in these cases, evidenced by their increased pulsation, while the symptoms referrible to the capillary circulation indicate rather unwonted activity than perversion of its natural functions: and in this case, as in that which has just been considered, it is evident that the unnatural accumulation and pressure of the affected blood-columns can only arise from one or both of two causes; viz. increased influx or diminished efflux. Either of these will clearly suffice for the production of the phenomena which constitute determination of blood; and I cannot understand why we should deny the possibility of the latter occasionally acting as well as the former cause. Whichever view we adopt, there can be little doubt that the principle determining that undue supply of blood to a particular artery which acts as the cause of various pathological phenomena, is, in the nature of the mechanism or contrivance by which it operates, identical with that regulating those variations in the distribution of the blood which are necessary for numerous physiological purposes. Before, then, we can clearly understand how a pathological determination of blood is induced, we must possess a precise knowledge of the nature and mode of operation of the immediate causes of the natural irregularities in the distribution of the circulating mass. And it is scarcely necessary to remark, that we have no positive information on this point. Dr. Billing is indeed the only writer who has even attempted a rational explanation of this action. He supposes that the coats of a particular artery, being weakened by the withdrawal of that nervous influence to which they owe their contractile power, oppose less resistance than natural to the distending pressure of the mass of aortic blood, an additional quantity of which is thus driven into that particular set of vessels. And though believing the contractility of the arterial tunics to be innate, and, therefore, not dependent upon a supply of nervous influence, I am by no means disposed to deny the possibility of their diminished contractile power, however induced, being occasionally the immediate cause of determination of blood. This view, it will be seen, refers the production of the local disorder of the circulation to an increased influx of blood consequent on the yielding of the coats of a particular artery. But it seems to me equally probable, that the same effect—the distension of the arterial ramifications by an unnatural accumulation of fluid—may result from an increased contraction of, and diminished efflux of blood from, the capillaries of the affected part. The immediate effect of this diminished rate of discharge from the capillaries must necessarily be an accumulation of blood in, and distension of, the more elastic and less contractile tubes situated behind the narrowed vessels; and in this manner the same phenomena will be induced as from the operation of the former cause. That contraction of the capillaries of the part is adequate to the causation of this pathological state, cannot be doubted, and various observations on the circulation show that a diminution in the size of the capillary streams does in some cases precede determination of blood: I allude to the phenomena witnessed on the application of stimuli to the transparent tissues of the lower animals; and the increased activity of the cutaneous circulation after *momentary* exposure to cold illustrates the operation of the same principle.

But though from physical reasoning it may be demonstrated that the increased lateral or distending pressure of the affected arterial columns can only arise from some change in the conditions regulating the discharge of blood into and from that system of tubes, it is advisable, in our present state of ignorance of the laws controlling the actions of the blood-vessels, to abstain from adopting either of these changes as the sole and invariable cause of determination of blood. The following tables exhibit the results of a few experiments which were undertaken for the purpose of elucidating some points connected with the pathology of this affection; and, though incapable of removing the difficulty which we have just been considering, they are not without some interest both in a physiological and pathological point of view.

From four young rabbits, of the same size and strength, the left kidney was removed through an incision in the loins, and immediately weighed. The animals were killed at different periods, and the weight of the remaining kidney and the condition of the urine carefully ascertained. The results were, that in—

TABLE IV.

Experiment.	The animal lived.	Left kidney weighed	Right kidney weighed.	The urine.
		Grains.	Grains.	
1	24 hours.	20	25	Contained no albumen.
2	3 days.	21	26	Ditto.
3	4 days.	20	33	Ditto.
4	9½ days.	21	50	Yielded a faint cloudiness with nitric acid.

A considerable number of observations would be required to enable us to determine with precision the average rate of increase in the size of the remaining organ. These few, however, suffice to show that it takes place gradually, and is—probably from that very circumstance—for the most part unaccompanied by any pathological phenomena. They also demonstrate the essentially vital nature of the process of arterial determination; for the closure of the left renal artery, as a *physical* cause, could have had very little to do with the enlargement of the right, its action (through the additional accumulation of blood in the aorta) being immediate; whereas the increased size of the latter vessel was clearly referrible to the operation of some slowly-acting persistent cause.

The next group of experiments exhibits the effects of an extreme and sudden increase in the supply of blood to an organ previously healthy. Having failed to produce any pathological phenomena, either by obstructing the aorta below the origin of the renal arteries, or by removing one kidney, I thought it possible that, by conjoining the two operations, and selecting stronger animals, more decided results might be obtained. In the paper published in the "Medico-Chirurgical Transactions for 1843," seven such experiments are related, in four of which the urine contained albuminous matters: but, as these successful experiments were not considered sufficiently numerous to counterbalance the failures, I have felt it necessary to repeat the observation, and trust that the additional facts now adduced will suffice to establish the point in question. The conditions of the experiment may be very briefly explained. In a strong and healthy animal, the aorta, exposed by an incision passing between the left lumbar and abdominal muscles, was completely obstructed, either by a ligature or by a small spring forceps, and the kidney on the same side then removed, its vessels being previously secured. The immediate effect of these measures would necessarily be an extreme accumulation of blood in the aorta, and a greatly increased supply to the vessels of the *right* kidney, which, of course, remained in its natural position, untouched and uninjured. The results are expressed in table V.*

TABLE V.

No. of experiment.	Weight of left kidney.	Weight of right kidney.	Difference in favour of right kidney.	Condition of urine.
	Grains.	Grains.	Grains.	
1*	30	30	0	Albuminous, and contained coagula of blood.
2*	35	42	7	Highly albuminous.
3*	82	112	30	Albuminous, and contained a fibrinous coagulum, and one of blood.
4*	54	85	31	Albuminous and bloody.
5	90	133	43	Stained with blood, but not distinctly albuminous.
6	123	130	7	Albuminous.
7	127	158	31	Highly albuminous.
8	118	152	34	Albuminous, and contained coagula of blood and fibrine.
9	94	150	56	Highly albuminous.
10	86	84	—	Albuminous, and contained a long narrow coagulum of blood, and several smaller ones.
11	Not ascertained.			Highly albuminous.
12	Notes lost.			Contained numerous minute coagula of blood.
13	144	150	6	Highly albuminous.

* The four first experiments on the list are those previously published; in the second, the occlusion of the aorta was not complete.

When the urine is described as simply albuminous it is to be inferred that there was no discoloration from any admixture of blood. The albuminous matters which it contained could only have been derived from the right kidney; for the left ureter was included in the same ligature with the blood-vessels of the left kidney at the time of removing that organ; and the existence of ecchymoses in the substance and on the surface of the remaining kidney, the presence of bloody and fibrinous coagula and of albuminous urine in the right ureter (as observed in Experiments 3, 7, and 9), and the fact of highly albuminous urine being, in the last-mentioned experiment, found in the right ureter, while the fluid taken from the bladder presented no albuminous impregnation, taken conjointly, render it impossible to doubt the accuracy of this statement.

These experiments, then, show that a *sudden and considerable* increase in the supply of blood to a part does occasion immediate pathological phenomena, in this respect differing materially from a slow and gradual determination of blood; and a comparison of the amount of increase in the weight of the remaining kidney with the nature of the effused matters will also prove that here, as after venous obstruction, there is no constant connection between these two circumstances; the only cause to which we can attribute the varieties noticed in the pathological effects being a difference in the degree of lateral pressure exercised by the impeded capillary blood-columns. This difference will, of course, mainly depend upon the activity of the circulation at the time of performing the experiment; but it is here interesting to inquire, how an increased flow of blood into a particular artery causes an unnatural amount of lateral pressure of the capillary streams supplied from that vessel. And an examination of this point is the more necessary, as it involves the solution of a pathological problem of some importance, viz. the *modus operandi* of determination of blood in inducing inflammation.

Whatever may be the action of its immediate cause, the pathological condition characterising determination of blood is undoubtedly an unnatural accumulation of that fluid in, and consequent distension of the arteries of, a particular part or organ; the blood columns contained within the minute porous capillaries of the affected part moving more rapidly than usual, and being therefore free from any material increase in their lateral or distending pressure. And as the facts and arguments adduced in the preceding part of this communication suffice, I think, to prove that inflammation is essentially constituted by an unnatural increase in the lateral pressure of the columns of blood contained within the *thin permeable capillaries*, the question may be reduced to a simpler form, and we shall merely have to inquire how a certain physical derangement of the arterial circulation in a particular part or organ is enabled to produce a similar affection of the capillaries continuous with the distended arteries.

The smaller arterial ramifications, in their healthy state, oppose a constant resistance to the distending pressure of the mass of blood pent up in the large arteries, and thus preserve the capillaries from an irruption of highly compressed fluid, which, if not at once structurally injurious, would be wholly subversive of their natural functions. But when this protection is, in a certain set of vessels, removed by the yielding of the smaller arteries, and the admission into them of an increased quantity of blood, the capillaries become directly exposed to the full force of the dilating columns. And if that lateral or dilating pressure be very great, or long continued, the opposing contractility of the capillaries becomes exhausted, and the accumulated and compressed blood, forcing an entrance into the debilitated vessels, rapidly occasions the pathological phenomena characteristic of inflammation. This view at once harmonises with, and explains, the fact of inflammation never supervening upon determination but when the latter disorder has been intense, frequent, or long continued. Since, then, the existence of an adequate distending force in the arterial blood-columns cannot be denied, and since the continued application of this hydraulic pressure must evidently have the effect of gradually and successively dilating the porous capillaries, and admitting into them a quantity of compressed blood, — conditions which, while incompatible with the discharge of the healthy functions of those vessels, are demonstrably productive of the pathological condition constituting inflammation, — it must be admitted that the occasioual appearance of this latter more serious disorder, as the effect of determination of blood, is clearly explicable by, and the result of, this physical process.

Another occasional effect of determination of blood is hæmorrhage, from the rupture of some of the distended arteries. This is of course most likely to occur when the arterial coats are diseased, or when the disorder affects vessels which are naturally weak; as in the brain.

But determination of blood sometimes produces a third effect, namely, the hypertrophy of the part thus unduly supplied. As we are at present merely inquiring into the nature, causation, and mode of operation of that disorder of the circulation, I cannot here enter upon the consideration of the circumstances which distinguish physiological from pathological hypertrophy. It may be sufficient to observe, that the physico-vital condition present, is in both cases the same. It is, however, necessary to mention the distinctions between hypertrophy and inflammation, as induced by determination of blood. These two states differ—1. In the relative intensity and duration of their immediate cause. Hypertrophy is the result of a slow, gradual, and continued increase in the supply of blood to a particular part, while a sudden and considerable increase in the influx of blood gives rise to the phenomena of inflammation. 2. The condition of the vessels of the affected part varies in the two cases. When determination of blood ends in inflammation, there is a considerable disproportion between the aggregate area of the capillaries of the affected part and that of the arteries supplying them; the former being in a greater or less portion of their extent contracted, unyielding, and thus rendered incapable of transmitting the blood accumulated in the former; while, in hypertrophy, both arteries and capillaries seem to dilate nearly in the same proportion, and the arterial blood being thus enabled rapidly to escape, the intensity of its pressure becomes very much diminished. And this circumstance enables us to understand how, 3rdly, hypertrophy and inflammation differ in their effects. In the former case, from the cause just mentioned, the lateral pressure of the blood entering the capillaries is very slightly increased, and a more active performance of the natural process of nutritive effusion is the only effect induced. This increased effusion may, in one part, furnish more material for a secretion; at other points it will supply the tissues with an unusual quantity of nutritive fluid; and when a gland is the organ unduly supplied with blood, both secretion and nutrition will proceed with inordinate activity. But in inflammation the lateral pressure of the capillary blood-columns is much increased, and it therefore presents, in its effects, a more marked deviation from their natural functions. The quantity of effused matter is more considerable, and instead of a solution of albumen, the fibrinous portion of the liquor sanguinis is also effused. As the processes of healthy or nutritive, and morbid or inflammatory effusion, are, however, both referrible to the same immediate cause, inflammation and hypertrophy virtually differ rather in degree than in nature; the greater intensity of the expelling pressure, and the more considerable extent of effusing surface present in the former affection, giving rise to its distinctive peculiarities.

It now only remains to consider the means by which the restoration to a natural state of the vessels affected in determination of blood is accomplished; and the examination of this question will at once conduct us to the principles on which its treatment is to be conducted.

From the remarks which have been made in explaining the production of its other terminations, it is evident that the local arterial hyperæmia which constitutes this disorder can only be removed by the contraction of the affected vessels, and the resumption and maintenance of their normal calibre. The removal, then, of every circumstance which can impede this reaction, and the employment of every measure which may appear calculated to facilitate and favour it, are clearly the two great principles to be observed in the treatment of this affection.

As regards the first point, the removal, where practicable, of the exciting cause and the diminution of the pressure of the fluid columns distending the affected vessels are the chief ends to be attempted. The former, as a general therapeutic rule, requires no comment: on the most advantageous method of effecting the latter object a few words may not be altogether useless. Determination of blood, like inflammation, may exist *with or without* general plethora; and in the treatment of both affections a constant reference to the quantity of circulating fluid is indispensable to successful practice. When, therefore, determination of blood exists with general plethora, in addition to other remedial measures, it will be found necessary to use depletion by means of blood-letting, purgation, &c., and to enforce low diet, in order to reduce and maintain at that diminished amount the *general* pressure of the arterial blood. But, on the other hand, where there is merely a *local* increase in the pressure of the arterial blood, and that referrible rather to the relaxation than to the forcible dilatation of the affected vessels, the equalisation of the circulation, by directing an additional quantity of blood to other and distant parts of the body, and thus diminishing the pressure upon the distended arteries, will sufficiently fulfil this indication. We accomplish this end by the use of derivatives, of which the best and most effectual, where it can with propriety be applied, is gentle and continued bodily exercise. In affections of particular organs, the derivation is variously directed. Thus, in determination of blood to the head, by a half instinctive feeling the supply to the lower extremities is artificially increased. When any internal organ becomes the seat of this disorder, by warmth or other stimulants the cutaneous vessels are stimulated so as to cause their enlargement. The general principle is, to determine either to the most distant parts, or to those which, from exercising a function similar to that of the affected organ, may, by their increased activity, diminish or remove the physiological necessity for its augmented supply of blood. The practice proposed by the late Dr. Parry of Bath, which consists in the compression of the arterial trunk leading to the seat of the determination, and which has been occasionally tried with success in this affection of the cerebral arteries, accomplishes directly what derivatives can only effect secondarily, namely, a diminution of the pressure acting upon the affected vessels. Its general impracticability is the only argument against its universal adoption.

The second indication in the treatment of this disorder is, to assist the arteries as much as possible in their reaction. In most cases we can only indirectly promote this salutary effort by withdrawing the distending force; but in determination to the head, the application of cold to the surface is found to exercise a direct action in favouring the contraction of the enlarged vessels. The influence of this agent is not confined to the capillaries; it is capable of diminishing the calibre of arteries of considerable size, whether immediately applied to them, or propagating its influence along the coats of the smaller vessels.

I have now endeavoured to trace the morbid effects resulting from an obstruction to the blood's passage through the different parts of the circulating system.

Venous obstruction is important chiefly from its disordering the capillary circulation. And such is the admirable arrangement adopted by nature for the prevention of this occurrence, that there are very few parts in which the closure of one vein will completely arrest, or even materially disturb, the circulation through the capillaries.

The importance of these disorders of the circulation

cannot be over estimated; for where they do not rapidly destroy life, they seldom fail to leave behind the material for structural change, and thus insidiously pave the way for numerous distressing and fatal maladies. In their earlier stages they are generally remediable; but the removal of the effects which result from their protracted continuance, or frequent recurrence, must ever be most difficult. Like many other diseases, their causes may be more easily removed than their effects.

Part VIII.

OF THE TREATMENT OF INFLAMMATION.

Among other advantages to be derived from the extension of our pathological knowledge is the substitution of an intelligible and scientific for a vague and empirical treatment of disease. Our ignorance of the nature and immediate causes of many morbid conditions will probably long compel us to employ remedial agents whose mode of operation is in a great measure equally obscure. But the superiority of a system of therapeutics in which it shall be possible to trace the chain of connection between the administration of the remedy and the removal of the disorder, must be sufficiently obvious.

Nor is the elucidation of the pathology of an affection practically useless, even where a tolerably successful plan of treatment has already been derived from a continued course of experimental observations on the diseased body, or, in other words, from empirical practice. For a knowledge of the essential nature and mode of action of the immediate causes of a disease, by exhibiting the circumstances which determine its varied degrees of intensity, naturally indicates corresponding modifications in its treatment, and thus regulates, by fixed and definite principles, points of practice which would otherwise be left wholly to the judgment of an individual. The advancement of pathology, therefore, not only tends directly to the extension and elevation of therapeutical science, by suggesting new measures for the prevention and removal of disease, but also enables us to command greater precision in the use of known remedies, by reducing into constant and intelligible laws the vague impressions and conflicting results of individual experience.

The measures found most successful in the treatment of inflammation are in such exact accordance with my conclusions as to the essential nature of that disease, that in a former part of this communication I could not avoid deducing, from their very efficacy, an argument in favour of the pathological doctrine there advanced. But, though experience has thus anticipated the results of reasoning, it may not be altogether uninteresting or uninstructive to present here a brief outline of the principles of treatment which are suggested by the foregoing views of the nature of that affection. This will, at any rate, enable the practitioner to compare the therapeutic rules thus obtained with those by which he is now influenced in the employment of the same remedies.

The first and chief principle to be observed in the treatment of inflammation, is the diminution of that unnatural pressure of the blood contained within the arteries and capillaries of the affected part which occasions its symptoms and immediate effects; while a second and scarcely less important indication has for its object the removal of those effects. And these two principles will be found to embrace everything of essential importance in the treatment of this affection. But simple as they may appear, their practical application will be found to require the exercise of no little skill and judgment in correctly proportioning the activity of the agents employed to the peculiar necessities of each case.

In the mode of action of its causes, and in the details of its treatment, acute inflammation differs so materially from those less intense forms of the disorder which are variously known as asthenic, passive, congestive, chronic, &c., that for practical purposes they may almost be regarded as two distinct diseases. And as it is impossible to consider separately the innumerable shades of intensity which inflammation presents, my remarks will chiefly have reference to well-marked examples of the sthenic and asthenic varieties of the complaint.

Acute inflammation is in general either the result of the application of some local irritant, or a consequence of determination of blood; its supervention upon the latter disorder being very frequently induced by the co-existence of a state of general plethora. As the disease under these circumstances originates rather in the arteries, than in the capillaries, of the affected part, an early and vigorous use of measures calculated to fulfil the first-mentioned therapeutic indication, will generally suffice for the restoration of the capillary circulation to its normal state. But when, as more frequently happens, the distending pressure of the accumulated blood has been permitted to act for a length of time upon the walls of the capillaries, the contractility of these vessels becomes gradually exhausted throughout the whole, or a great portion, of their extent; they cease to oppose any *active* resistance to the dilating force of the contained fluid columns; the effusion of fibrinous and albuminous matter, or the extravasation of blood, proceeds uninterruptedly, and a tedious and probably imperfect recovery is the most favourable result which can be expected.

Before, however, considering at greater length the principles which should regulate the employment of the more active antiphlogistic remedies, a few words on the diagnosis of internal inflammation may not be altogether misplaced. For every careful and candid practitioner must have occasionally experienced the difficulty of distinguishing between cases of real and merely apparent inflammation, and will also admit the *possibility* of inflammatory disease proceeding in a vital organ to a dangerous and even fatal extent, without occasioning, during its progress, any perceptible morbid phenomena. Nor does the existence of these difficulties appear extraordinary when we reflect upon the uncertainty and inconclusiveness of many of the data to which we are compelled to trust for the detection of disease. The power of correctly appreciating the value of symptoms is one of the highest qualifications of a medical practitioner; but this faculty, in its highest and most perfect form, can be acquired only by an attentive study of the laws of life as contained in the sciences of physiology and pathology. And I cannot but think that a neglect of this important study, consequent on an unreflecting and lasting adoption of the dogmatic, and in many instances unfounded, statements and unmeaning definitions of systematic nosologists, has been productive of some serious errors, both in the diagnosis and treatment of disease. These writers seem to have frequently mistaken its symptoms or effects for the disease itself, and by thus confounding, in their own minds, certain generally co-existent but non-essential phenomena with the actual malady, they have naturally impressed others with an idea that the two are inseparable, and consequently that the presence of these phenomena constitutes satisfactory proof of the existence of the disease: whereas, it is now generally admitted that the number of really pathognomonic symptoms is very limited; that the same morbid sensations and unnatural appearances may result from very opposite causes, and require for their removal very different plans of treatment, and that in the diagnosis of disease it is more prudent to check our first impressions until they have been tested and verified by a careful and comprehensive review of the great functions of the body, than to rely implicitly upon one or more prominent local symptoms.

Now, local pain, a very general and by far the most striking symptom of internal inflammation, is, if taken *per se*, perhaps the most fallacious of all the manifestations of disordered action, for it may not only exist with the most opposite states of the system, and even with very different local disorders of the circulation, but being regulated in its severity chiefly by the degree of sensibility possessed by the particular constitution or part affected, it ceases to furnish any definite information as to the activity or danger, or even the nature of the existing malady. The diseases, therefore, most liable to be mistaken for acute inflammation, are those in which the sensibility of a part or organ is, from some other cause, unnaturally augmented; such are neuralgic, hysterical, and rheumatic pains, and also certain forms of cerebral excitement. The special rules for discriminating between it and these several affections are, of course, inadmissible in a sketch of the general pathology of inflammation; but in addition to the other precautions already noticed I may mention the propriety of instituting, where practicable, a physical examination of the part affected, and of ascertaining, by the application of chemical agents, the nature of any change which may have taken place in the fluid discharged by glandular or effusing surfaces. The age, sex, diathesis, habits, &c. of the individual will also materially assist the diagnosis.

Certain peculiar states of the constitution may moreover give rise to symptoms very closely resembling those of acute inflammation. In persons of a debilitated habit, in whom there exists at the same time great irritability of the nervous system—a combination of frequent occurrence in women and children—there may often be observed a tendency to morbid excitement of the nerves of sensation, very similar to that described by Dr. Hall and others, as one of the occasional effects of loss of blood. But of all the forms of pseudo-inflammatory disease, that simulation of peritonitis occasionally met with in the puerperal state is the most perplexing. Every symptom of inflammation may then be present; there may be a considerable degree of fever, quickness, and some hardness of the pulse, with intense pain (not confined merely to the skin covering the peritoneum), and the disease will nevertheless often rapidly vanish under the use of fomentations, alteratives, and moderate purgation. The task of determining the inflammatory or non-inflammatory nature of affections presenting the most prominent symptoms of that disease, is therefore occasionally one of the greatest difficulty. And an error on this point, whether leading to the reduction of a system already too much enfeebled, or to the toleration, if not the active encouragement, of acute inflammatory disease, has doubtless often been productive of very lamentable consequences.

The necessity of distinguishing between chronic inflammation and other lingering internal ailments is less urgent than when the disease assumes a more active form. It is also less practicable: but as the treatment of most chronic internal affections presents many points of resemblance, the probability of any serious error arising from its confusion with other disorders is very much diminished.

Resuming, then, the consideration of the principles on which the treatment of acute inflammation is to be conducted, let us examine the action of the remedies calculated to effect the first mentioned indication; namely, the diminution of the unnatural pressure of the blood contained within the vessels of the affected part. It has already been explained that the amount of distending pressure exercised by the blood detained in the obstructed capillaries is mainly regulated by the degree of impulse imparted to each minute arterial column by the pressure of the great mass of aortic blood. By reducing the general pressure of the blood contained within the arterial system, we therefore necessarily diminish the lateral pressure of the blood accumulated behind the obstructed portion of the affected capillaries, and thus relieve the intensity of the symptoms and reduce the activity of the inflammatory attack. The measures by which we are enabled to accomplish this object are very numerous; and the relative permanency of their depressing influence upon the system varying much, a wide field is left for the skill of the practitioner to exercise itself in selecting those best adapted to the peculiar circumstances of each case.

We reduce the general pressure of the arterial blood—

1. By diminishing the quantity of the circulating fluid;

2. By reducing the force and frequency of the heart's action.

The quantity of the circulating fluid may be diminished —

1. By the direct abstraction of blood;
2. By draining off its aqueo-albuminous portion;
3. By abstinence from nourishment.

Now the propriety of restricting the supply of food to the lowest possible amount in cases of acute inflammation is unquestionable; nor can there be much difference of opinion as to the beneficial effect which generally attends a diminution of the quantity and impulse of the circulating fluid by means of active purgatives, diaphoretics, &c. But the abstraction of any considerable quantity of blood, and particularly the repetition of such a step, should always be preceded by a careful examination of the peculiarities of the constitution under treatment, and a comparison of them with the laws regulating the employment of that powerful agent.

Blood-letting is frequently so convenient a remedy, and the temporary relief which it affords from painful and distressing symptoms so immediate and certain, that a hasty and unreflecting practitioner may insensibly contract a habit of using it where milder measures would prove equally efficacious. It moreover carries with it an appearance of vigour and promptness in the treatment of the complaint which is in general far from displeasing to the patient and his friends, and, through its powerful sedative influence on the system, it for a time so completely removes the unpleasant sensations, which in the mind of the sufferer constitute his disease, that its repetition is sometimes actually solicited. This very valuable remedy, is therefore, like many others, from a variety of causes, liable to be abused. And while admitting the great advantage which attends copious blood-letting in many, perhaps a majority of cases of acute inflammation, I cannot avoid entertaining an opinion that, notwithstanding the judicious advice which has been offered by various writers, and the forcible description given by Dr. Hall of the injurious consequences of excessive or protracted loss of blood, the treatment of inflammation is still occasionally characterised by a great disregard of the evils which may result from an incautious use of the measures employed for its removal.

With the exception of cases in which the importance of the organ or part affected is such as to compel us to overlook the dangers and disadvantages which may result from the subsequent debility, general blood-letting seems to me to be chiefly and almost solely applicable to individuals in whom inflammation has supervened on, and exists with, a state of general plethora. Under these circumstances the quantity of circulating fluid is not only excessive, but the proportion of its fibrinous constituent is also unnaturally augmented; and a free abstraction of blood, by venesection or otherwise, then acts beneficially by changing the quality, as well as by diminishing the quantity and impulse, of the circulating mass. But where there is no reason to suspect any material disorder in the quality or abnormal increase in its quantity,—as when the disease is referrible to some local irritation, or occurs in persons of nervous and excitable constitution,—depressants, the influence of which upon the system is less permanent than that of blood-letting, will generally be found capable of fulfilling every useful purpose served by that remedy. We see every immediate effect of venesection to follow the administration of powerful purgatives, nauseants, and sedatives; we know that they rapidly diminish the quantity of the circulating fluid, reduce the force and frequency of the heart's action, and allay the general irritability produced by the local disorder; and why then should we, except under particular circumstances and for special reasons, such as those above-mentioned, subject our patients to the protracted debility, not to mention the possible danger, of general blood-letting? By administering in the first instance powerful and rapidly-acting purgatives, and then keeping the system for a time under the depressing influence of antimony or mercury, or using with these remedies still more direct sedatives, such as tobacco and digitalis, we may frequently obtain the beneficial effects, without encountering the disadvantages, resulting from a large loss of blood.

In making these observations, I am far from attempting to dispute the great value of a free use of the lancet in many cases of acute inflammation: I merely object to its indiscriminate employment in all forms of the disease, to its adoption as an item of routine practice. And the great evils attending a practical neglect or forgetfulness of the previous existence and operation, in many individuals, of various debilitating causes, such as poverty, residence in large towns or in unwholesome dwellings, sedentary occupations, dissipated habits, &c. may perhaps excuse and justify this brief allusion to the subject.

The local measures by which the unnatural pressure of the obstructed capillary blood-columns is relieved are—

1. The escape of a portion of the compressed blood through apertures occasioned either naturally, by their rupture from excessive distension, or artificially, by acupuncture, incisions, leeches, &c.;

2. The escape of the liquor sanguinis through the pores of the capillaries;

3. The use of derivatives,

In some forms of acute inflammation, as in gastritis and other cases in which a mucous membrane is the seat of the disease, the morbidly increased lateral pressure of the accumulated blood is sometimes spontaneously relieved by free hæmorrhage, the result of the rupture of the distended vessels. But it is, of course, only in certain inflammatory affections of the superficial structures of the body that it is possible to imitate, by punctures and scarifications, this natural method of cure.

The effusion of the more liquid portion of the blood through the pores of the distended vessels relieves the intensity of the compression of the detained fluid almost as completely as its escape *en masse*. And for the sake of obtaining that present relief, effusion is perhaps too frequently encouraged by the local application of warmth and moisture. Now, when it is remembered that every atom of the effused matter must be absorbed before a perfect cure can be effected, it is, I think, almost a self-evident proposition that, in general, the effusion should be limited to the smallest possible amount; and, where practicable, should be altogether prevented. Were it not for the difficulties which we encounter in attempting to accomplish the removal of the local effects of inflammation, our treatment of it would always be certain and rapidly successful: for we could in every instance soon relieve the intensity of the blood's pressure in the affected vessels. But the absorption of any considerable quantity of extravasated liquor sanguinis is invariably a work of time; and where the fibrinous portion has become firmly coagulated or at all organised, our most potent remedies, in the hands of the most skilful practitioner, will often fail to relieve the adjacent structures of the substances thus forced amongst them. There is, therefore, every inducement to prevent as far as possible the occurrence of any sanguineous or fibrinous infiltration of the tissues of the affected part.

Effusion is, however, sometimes very useful as a derivative agent, where it can with propriety be obtained from vessels situated at a little distance from, but communicating freely with, those which are the seat of the inflammatory disorder. And a good instance of its beneficial operation under these circumstances is presented in the success attending the early administration of purgatives in peritonitis.

The results of medical practice here harmonise very beautifully with some experimental observations (related in Magendie's Journal), in which, on exposing and irritating a fold of mesentery, the redness caused by the enlargement and distension of the peritoneal vessels rapidly disappeared when free effusion took place from the adjacent mucous membrane. And the mode of action of all other derivatives, such as leeches, cupping, blisters, &c., in relieving the engorgement of the affected vessels, is precisely similar. If, however, any considerable quantity of blood or serum be thus abstracted, it will, of course, in addition to its local action, also tend to diminish the general pressure of the arterial blood. It is scarcely necessary to add, that effusion as a derivative agent is admissible only in situations where the arrangement of the vessels is such as to allow of a free discharge and ready removal of the extravasated matters: in the use of counter-irritants we are therefore necessarily restricted to the skin and mucous membranes.

Having thus reviewed the operation of the remedies calculated to relieve that local disorder of the circulation which constitutes the essence of inflammation, we have in the next place to consider the means by which the removal of the immediate effects of that disease is accomplished. But, before entering upon this subject, it may be observed, that we occasionally have it in our power to prevent, or at least limit, by the direct application of mechanical support, the escape of the compressed fluid through the coats of the distended vessels. Effusion, as before mentioned, can only occur when the pressure acting on the internal surface of the minute porous vessels, preponderates over that operating on their exterior. By artificially increasing the amount of this latter force, at the same time that we diminish the lateral pressure of the obstructed blood-columns, we are therefore often enabled to exercise a direct as well as an indirect influence in checking the process of effusion. And in inflammatory affections of the superficial structures and organs of the body, where pressure can be directly applied, an observance of this principle will sometimes materially expedite the recovery.

In discussing the various questions connected with the nature of inflammation, I more than once had occasion to enumerate its immediate effects, the removal of which, next to the alleviation of the morbid state itself, constitutes the chief object of our treatment. The physiological action most concerned in this restorative process is vascular absorption, or that function by means of which fluids, placed in contact with the external surface of the blood-vessels, traverse their coats, and so enter and mingle with the mass of circulating blood. In the application of our remedies during this stage of the treatment, we have therefore to attempt—1st, to facilitate and assist, by every means in our power, the absorbing process; and 2ndly, to promote the solution of such effused matters as may have become solidified, and so render them capable of absorption.

Before, however, this physiological process can be employed with much success or certainty as a remedial agent, we must possess a clear and definite knowledge of the seat, the active cause, and the mechanism of absorption. And on these points there exists among physiologists some difference of opinion.

The doctrine now generally received, both in this country and on the continent, is that advanced by Magendie and others, who refer the act of absorption to an affinity of the vascular walls for the matters absorbed; the absorbing power of the capillary membrane being, in their opinion, assisted by the unequal density and viscidity of the fluids situated on either surface. Against this doctrine I have, on a former occasion, advanced various objections: amongst others—

1. That the laws of endosmosis and exosmosis apply only to stagnant fluids, and not to rapidly-moving streams, like those traversing the capillaries.

2. That it does not explain how, in certain parts of the body, one or other action, namely, either effusion or absorption, wholly preponderates.

3. That the force which it supposes to operate is not sufficiently active to cause that rapid absorption which we so often witness.

4. That it leaves us as ignorant as before of the immediate cause of absorption, and is therefore practically useless in guiding our employment of that process as a remedial agent.

Conceiving, therefore, that neither the porosity of the capillary walls nor the difference in the physical properties of the fluids situated on either surface of that membrane, constituted a satisfactory explanation of the mechanism of absorption, I proceeded to inquire how far *the motion of the blood* might be employed as the active cause of this important process; and, from an examination of the general absorbing power possessed by all moving fluids, and a comparison of the physical conditions most favourable to the operation of this power with those regulating the passage of the blood through the cylindrical capillaries and adjacent venous radicles, I considered myself justified in advancing an opinion "that the active power employed in the animal body for the performance of absorption, resides in the currents of blood which incessantly traverse the veins and terminating portion of the capillaries.* "

The grounds on which I am for the present content to rest this opinion may be thus enumerated:—

1. It is an established physical law that all freely-moving currents exercise an absorbing power, or, in other words, draw with them any stagnant fluid with which they may directly or indirectly come in contact; this power being proportioned to the rapidity of their motion.

2. It is an evident fact that the streams of blood do traverse the minute blood-vessels with very great velocity.

3. The anatomical arrangement of the terminating portion of the capillaries, and the conditions regulating the passage of the blood through the veins, are such as to facilitate the motion, and consequently, increase the absorbing power, of the minute blood-currents.

* Medical Gazette, 1844.

4. The tenuity and porosity of the capillary walls being also demonstrable, it must be admitted as perfectly possible for the freely-moving streams traversing those minute vessels to exercise, through the intervening pores, their power of lateral draught upon any external stagnant fluid.

As this doctrine refers absorption to the motion of the blood, as its direct and active cause, we are by it at once enabled to understand why absorption invariably ceases as soon as the circulation through a part is arrested,—a fact established by numerous experiments. And, as the absorbing power of the minute blood-streams operates by diminishing the pressure acting on the internal surface of the capillaries, it is moreover in perfect harmony with those observations of Magendie, in which he found the rapidity of the absorbing process to be increased by vascular depletion. The mode of operation of this important law is indeed rendered more intelligible by it than by the general doctrine of absorption propounded by that illustrious physiologist himself.

It will be seen that the essential difference between the opinion of Magendie on the mechanism of absorption, and that which I have ventured to advance, consists in this circumstance—that, whereas he considers the active power employed in this process to reside in the capillary membrane, and that the streams of blood merely carry away the fluids which that membrane has absorbed, I claim for the rapidly moving blood-columns the chief, the prime, the active share in the operation, and regard the intervening membrane as perfectly passive, contributing nothing more than its porosity towards the performance of the function. The power of lateral draught exercised by freely-moving streams has been mentioned by various writers on Natural Philosophy, as probably assisting the circulation through some of the communicating venous branches; but I am not aware of any other physiologist having adduced it in explanation of the mechanism of absorption, by supposing it to act through the pores situated in the capillary walls upon any external fluids.*

In order, then, to obtain the absorption of the matters effused during inflammation, we must in every case increase, as far as possible, the *general* absorbing power of the capillary blood-currents, while we at the same time apply, wherever practicable, local remedies, calculated either to augment the pressure acting on the exterior of the affected vessels, or to promote the activity of the circulation through them. The first object is accomplished by a persistence in the use of evacuants, and by continning to limit the quantity of ingesta; the effect of this diminution of the bulk of the circulating mass being a more free and unimpeded passage of the blood through the capillaries, whereby both the activity of the absorbing process, and the extent of

* Dr. C. J. B. Williams, in his Principles of Medicine, page 271, represents me as having illustrated, by some experiments, views on absorption advanced by him in his Gulstonian lectures; the substance of which appeared in the "Medical Gazette" (July, 1841). I have carefully examined the communications referred to, but have failed to discover in them any opinion on the nature or mechanism of absorption differing from that of Magendie.

absorbing surface are materially increased. Some of the chief *local* measures by which we endeavour to aid the natural powers of absorption in the affected part have been already alluded to as useful in preventing effusion. Such are the application of cold and astringents, mechanical support, by means of bandaging, strapping, &c. To these may now be added friction, which, however, when employed for this purpose, should not be confined to the mere surface of the skin. A gentle, continued, kneading pressure, following the course of the venous blood, is much more efficacious, and, in some forms of subcutaneous effusion, exercises a marked influence in accelerating the removal of serous fluid. Blisters, and various internal remedies, used for the dispersion of the immediate effects of inflammation, seem to me to operate rather by promoting the solution of the effused and solidified fibrine than by contributing any direct aid to the absorbing process.

It is evident that any measures which tend to remove the products of effusion by adding to, and co-operating with, the natural powers of absorption, can be successful so long only as those matters retain a certain degree of fluidity: for the passage of a mass of solid fibrine through the minute pores of the capillary membrane is clearly a physical impossibility. Now, whilst in the transparent gelatinous state, which it retains for some time after its effusion, the fibrine of the liquor sanguinis is, I believe, capable of very rapid absorption. And, in support of this opinion, I may mention an experiment, performed by me some years since, in which a quantity of extremely tenacious semi-gelatinous ov-albumen, very similar in physical appearance to recently effused fibrine, was introduced into the peritoneum of a rabbit; and on killing and examining the animal a few hours afterwards, not a particle of it was to be found. In the treatment of inflammation we have, therefore, every inducement to be prompt and vigorous in the use of remedies calculated to accelerate the absorbing process, inasmuch as the delay of a few hours may convert a semi-fluid mass, capable of speedy absorption, into a solid unmanageable substance, which, prior to the possibility of its removal, must undergo a tedious and uncertain process of digestion.

It is not my intention to dwell at any length upon the action of the particular remedies by which we endeavour to promote the absorption of solidified fibrine. The preparations of mercury and of iodine, and the alkaline salts, which are the substances generally administered in these cases, can but indirectly assist absorption by aiding the solution of the effused matters. The relative power of these agents, and the conditions under which they operate with greater activity, are points on which we do not possess much positive information, and from their great practical importance, it is highly desirable that they should be made the subject of further investigation.

We have now noticed the two chief principles to be observed in the treatment of acute inflammation. Were it possible by any medicinal agencies to directly remove the capillary obstruction, which constitutes the immediate cause of the disease, the early adoption of such measures would, of course, be imperatively called for. But as the attainment of this object is, in the majority of cases, clearly impossible, we are compelled to limit our efforts to the prevention and removal of the injurious effects resulting from the existence of that local impediment to the circulation. Most of the remedies, however, employed for this purpose also exercise a considerable influence in accelerating the disintegration and softening of the coagulated blood-columns, and thus facilitate the re-establishment of the circulation through the affected vessels. Some of those just mentioned as useful in promoting the removal of the solid products of effusion, have more especially been long celebrated for their *deobstruent* powers.

As the first stage of inflammation, or that characterised by effusion, ceases with the solidification of the columns of blood occupying the affected vessels, and as the present inquiry is not intended to embrace the study of more than that stage of the disease, I shall not further pursue the examination of the treatment of its acute forms. In accordance with the plan laid down at its commencement, I have throughout this investigation studiously avoided any discussion of the many important circumstances which determine the nature of the secondary effects of inflammation. And from the same desire to exclude, as far as possible, all sources of complication, even those more obvious chemico-physical peculiarities of the circulating fluid, which tend to modify its immediate and primary effects, have been passed over in silence. I repeat this explanation, because I might otherwise be supposed to recognise, in all cases of inflammation, none other than the purely physical disorder of the blood, which arises from the local obstruction to its passage through the capillaries.

The preceding remarks have had reference solely to the treatment of acute or sthenic inflammation; but, before dismissing the subject, it is necessary to make a few observations upon the management of the opposite forms of the disease. Chronic inflammation, whether occurring primarily, or as the effect of an acute inflammatory attack, is invariably connected with a relaxed condition of the affected vessels; and this impaired tone of the capillaries of the part is, in the former class of cases, generally complicated with a debilitated state of the constitution. Although, therefore, this complaint undoubtedly presents a tendency to effusion indicative of an unnatural increase in the lateral pressure of the retarded blood-columns, our attention must here be fixed rather upon the defective tone of the contractile tissues which occasions that local retardation of the circulation, than upon the physical disorder of the blood resulting from its existence. The pathology of this form of the disease is, indeed, correctly represented by that doctrine of inflammation which refers its causation to a relaxation of the coats of the capillaries, followed by an accumulation and tendency to coagulation of the impeded blood. And the existence of the slight impeding cause constituted by that extreme capillary relaxation, will necessarily tend to induce and maintain, throughout the whole extent of the affected vessels, a constant but moderate lateral pressure of the detained fluid; sufficient to occasion its partial exudation through the porous capillaries, without, at the same time, morbidly exciting the sensibility of the part.

In accordance, then, with these views of the nature and causation of the disorder, the chief object of our treatment must evidently be the re-invigoration of the affected vessels, and, if necessary, of the whole system; and, by the adoption of this course, the physical disorder of the enlarged and retarded columns of blood will in general be effectually removed, and its effects obviated. The treatment of asthenic inflammation is, therefore, based upon a precisely opposite principle to that which claims our chief attention in the management of the acute disease. In the latter, the power of the heart, and the resulting pressure or impulse of the arterial blood being very considerable, our first step is to diminish the amount of that pressure by the use of debilitating agents, and thus prevent any serious local injury resulting from the extravasation of blood, or effusion of liquor sanguinis. But in the primarily chronic or asthenic forms of the disease, the lateral pressure of the detained blood is comparatively inconsiderable; and though it may, in certain situations, be productive of copious serous effusion, or even fibrinous exudation, there never can be the same necessity for, nor will the system endure, anything like the active depletory measures demanded in cases of acute inflammation. There is, in short, this essential difference in the causation of these two varieties of inflammatory disease, that in the one form—the sthenic or acute—the debility or relaxation of the capillaries of the affected part is *an effect* of the physical disorder, or morbidly increased latêral pressure of the contained blood; while in chronic inflammation, occurring as a primary disease, the relaxation of the capillaries, by constituting a slight impediment to the blood's passage through them, operates as *the cause* of the accompanying physical disorder of that fluid. In treating this latter disease, we must, therefore, rather address ourselves to the removal of the primary obstructing cause, the relaxation of the affected capillaries (which is fortunately, to a great extent, remediable), than seek, by depletory measures, to relieve the accompanying physical disorder of the blood, which is but an effect of that obstruction.

The means by which we attempt to restore to their natural condition the relaxed capillaries, consist either in the direct application of astringents, stimulants, or mechanical support, or in the administration of remedies calculated to give tone to the whole system.

The employment of local remedies is, of course, necessarily restricted to those cases in which the disease affects structures situated near to the surface of the body. But where they can be used, as in affections of the conjunctiva, of the throat, of the rectal, vaginal, and urethral mucous membranes, and of the cutaneous and subcutaneous structures, their beneficial influence in expediting and frequently completing the recovery is daily exemplified. In the majority of cases of chronic inflammation, and particularly in those forms of it which occur idiopathically, and not from the application of any local irritant, it will, however, be found necessary to adopt measures having for their object the improvement of the general health, and the restoration of their natural vigour or tone to the contractile tissues of the body: and, as a preliminary step, it is in these cases always advisable to search for, with the view of removing, any debilitating causes to which each individual may have been particularly subject. For not only are the *general* causes of debility already sufficiently numerous, and (from the miserable and half-civilized condition of a large proportion of the population, and the want of proper social legislation) apparently on the increase, but each class of the community is more especially exposed to certain influences peculiar to itself. On the present occasion it is, of course, impossible to do more than allude to these injurious agencies, but it may be observed that they all involve a partial deprivation of one or more of those essentials to health which have long been pointed out by medical writers, and the chief of which are pure air, regular exercise, a sufficiency of wholesome nourishment, and the means of maintaining the natural temperature of the body.

Having, then, attended to those circumstances of diet and regimen, without which the administration of medicines will be of little avail, we may proceed to give such tonics as the state of the constitution more particularly demands. And here great advantage will be experienced from a knowledge of the peculiar diathesis of the individual, and of the nature and cause of any derangement in the quality of the blood. If there be merely an impoverished condition of the circulating fluid, a generous diet, assisted by chalybeates and aromatic tonics, will generally suffice for its restoration to a healthy state. And in cases where the relaxation of the capillaries, and the tenuity of the blood, are so extreme as to cause copious fluxes, or extensive serous effusions, these measures may be joined with the internal administration of astringents, such as the mineral acids or acetate of lead.

If, on the other hand, from the appearance of the individual, from the structure affected, and from the history of the case, we have reason to suspect a tendeney to the exudation of scrofulous matter, more benefit may perhaps be experienced from administering, instead of, or in addition to the other remedies, some preparation of iodine or any other substance that may appear calculated either to prevent the formation, or facilitate the removal, of that diseased albumen. So, likewise, in cases of rheumatic, syphilitic, and erysipelatous inflammation, must our treatment embrace as its chief object the removal of the peculiar disorder of the constitution, or of the blood, which originates and maintains the local disease.

In this brief sketch of the treatment of chronic inflammation nothing has been said of the use of counter-irritants or of local blood-letting; where this latter remedy can with propriety be adopted, the case must present more of a sthenic character than those which we have lately been considering, and in its treatment we must therefore be guided by the same principles which regulate the management of the more acute forms of the disease. And, as regards counter-irritation, a remedy of very great utility in the treatment of internal or deep-seated chronic inflammation, the benefit resulting from its employment is often so much greater than can be explained by its purely physical action as a derivative, that we are, I think, almost compelled to adopt, to a certain extent, the ancient idea that these artificial sores act as drains for the discharge of vitiated fluid from the blood.

These, then, appear to me to be the general principles on which the treatment of inflammation is to be conducted; and they are, I think, in perfect unison with what we know of the nature and causation of that disease. The extent to which, in each particular case, depressing or strengthening measures are to be pursued, must, of course, be left wholly to the judgment of the practitioner; and the greatest care and circumspection are in some cases required to enable us to arrive at a satisfactory conclusion on this important question. In applying to practical purposes the pathological views contained in the preceding part of this communication, I have, therefore, ventured to dissent in toto from those who think that all cases of inflammation are to be treated on *antiphlogistic* principles.

There doubtless still remain for investigation some obscure points connected with the nature and mode of action of the exciting causes of inflammation; and, as regards the peculiar circumstances which determine the production of its secondary effects, we may be said to know nothing with certainty. But as these questions, though constituting interesting and important ramifications from the general subject, need not necessarily be mixed up with an inquiry into the essential nature of inflammation, I have, on the present occasion, refrained as much as possible from entering upon their consideration.

The pathological views now advanced are, to a considerable extent, based upon those views of the physiology of the circulation which formed the subject of a former paper. There has, indeed, long existed an impression among those who have studied the actions of the living body, that the minute arteries effuse, and the venous radicles absorb: but, with the exception of that previously alluded to, no attempt has been made to discover the mechanism of either process, nor has the fact itself been established either by actual observation or physical reasoning. The former proof, though perhaps some day attainable, is not yet capable of being exhibited. But a judicious application of the principles of hydraulics to the explanation of the functions of the minute blood-vessels, does, I think, justify us in concluding that, during the existence of the circulation, a slow but constant *extravascular current* is, as a general rule, everywhere flowing from the arterial to the venous portion of the capillaries, and thus effects the nutrition and purification of the different tissues of the body.

To some these ideas may perhaps appear too purely mechanical; but they are not more so than that which, supported by similar principles of reasoning, enabled Harvey to anticipate the evidence of the senses. And, for my own part, I cannot understand how any doctrine can be *too* chemical, or *too* mechanical, *if it be but true.* No one can wish to introduce the spirit of sectarianism into science; and, as nature will neither change nor suspend her laws to suit our prejudices, it behoves us, before rejecting any new views on an obscure but important question, to advance against them some stronger argument than their mere antagonism to, or incongruity with, received opinions.

But the adoption of these views by no means implies the recognition of an exclusively mechanical system of physiology; for no one can be more willing than myself to confess the immensity of the distinction between living and dead matter, or to admit that the minutely-varied physical and vital endowments which characterise the different component tissues of each animal body, can only originate in a *creative* power infinitely superior to the laws regulating the phenomena of the inorganic world.

Any attempt at dispelling the darkness which has so long obscured the physiology and pathology of the circulation must, in a great measure, be necessarily founded upon physical reasoning; and, as all physiologists are not even yet prepared to admit that the motion of the blood is a purely mechanical action, it is not wonderful that, at the end of two centuries, our knowledge of its uses, and of the diseases which result from its derangement, should continue to be very imperfect. May we not, indeed, still say, with an intelligent physician of the last century—"It must be confessed that the discovery of the circulation has not been followed by so great advancement in the science of medicine as was naturally to have been expected from it. The reason of which is, that our theory has not yet advanced much in the knowledge which is naturally founded upon this grand principle—*the circulation.* It has not yet explained the epicycles, as I may be allowed to call the partial systems and various relations of parts, both fluid and solid, on which the anomalies of the body, the nature of diseases, and the operation of medicines, must depend. Had Newton only discovered the general operation of gravity upon all matter, and barely hinted that the motion of the planets must depend upon it, philosophers had then understood the system of the world nearly as well as we do now the system of the body."*

The want of zeal thus manifested in the study of perhaps the most beautiful phenomenon in nature, and certainly the most important action of the living animal, will doubtless excite the astonishment of after ages; and it were well for mankind if the causes which have thus retarded the growth of medical *science* were no longer in operation. The truth would seem to be, that, notwithstanding all the

* An Epistle to the Rev. Dr. Hales, introductory to an Essay on the Blood, by Richard Davies, M.D.: Bath, 1759.

praise and honours which have been heaped upon Harvey's name and memory, his principles of philosophy have never been really popular. Nor is this at all inexplicable, when we, on the one hand, consider the influence which fashion exercises in enconraging or discouraging certain lines of investigation; and observe, on the other, the very slight connection between devotion to the science of medicine, and success in its pursuit as a profession. Even the scanty information now possessed on this subject (much of which is but a revival of old opinions) has been chiefly obtained by the labour of Continental physiologists, and more especially of that illustrious school which owns Magendie as its founder. Nor, with the exception of Hales (a clergyman), can any of Harvey's fellow-countrymen be said to have materially contributed to the illustration and extension of his grand principle. And yet what other field of inquiry offers an equal prospect of obtaining brilliant and important results? The nature of the intimate connection shown by experiments to exist between the circulation of the blood and the manifestation of the higher functions of the nervous system, the dependence of calorification, and of the various purifying actions of the body upon the incessant continuance of that motion,—these and many other problems, the solution of which would be equally interesting and useful, all call for investigation. And who can take upon him to declare that the laws which regulate those phenomena will for ever remain inaccessible to patient observation, assisted by experiment, and conducted by strict, unprejudiced reasoning, to the establishment of sound and logical conclusions? Nor has anatomy yet ceased to unfold the varied structural arrangements by means of which nature is enabled to produce with one cause an infinity of effects; for every year brings with it an account of some minute mechanism, some beautiful contrivance, each admirably adapted, by means the most simple, to the accomplishment of ends the most elaborate and important. And who can say how many more such which the eye of man hath not yet seen, and all the uses of which the understanding of man shall perhaps never fully comprehend, may still exist, buried and concealed in the dark nooks and unexplored recesses of the animal body?

While meditating, then, upon the immeasurable benefits which his discovery would ultimately confer upon mankind, and thus gathering by anticipation the glory which would redound from it upon himself, his profession, and his country, well might Harvey exclaim, in a burst of lofty and almost prophetic enthusiasm—"Denique in omni parte medicinæ, physiologicâ, pathologicâ, semeioticâ, therapeuticâ, cum quot problemata determinari possint, ex hac datâ veritate et luce, quanta dubia solvi et quot obscura dilucidari, animo mecum reputo, campum invenio spatiosissimum, ubi longius percurrere et latins expatiari adeo possum, ut non solum in volumen excresceret, præter institutum meum, hoc opus, sed mihi forsan vita ad finem faciendum deficeret."*

* De motu cordis, cap. xvi.

ON THE

PATHOLOGICAL CHANGES OCCURRING IN CERTAIN DEVITALISED TISSUES.

[Communicated to the Royal Medical-Chirurgical Society of London. Received May 23rd, 1854; read June 27th, 1854.]

THE subordination of ordinary chemical laws to the superior controlling power of life, is one of the most interesting and important principles of physiology; and modern pathology is now rapidly establishing the converse of this proposition by demonstrating that the partial or complete destruction of their inherent vital powers again subjects to the general laws of matter the structures thus morbidly affected. Till a comparatively recent period, the various forms of *gangrene* were alone considered indicative of the death of a part; afterwards, *softening* of certain internal organs was pronounced an analogous pathological condition; and of late, the *degenerations* of tissues are admitted, by the best pathologists, to indicate and follow an insidious local deprivation of vital properties and powers in which many of the most fatal diseases originate.

When, therefore, from any cause, the tissues of the living body lose their vitality, either wholly or in part, they at once begin to undergo processes of degeneration and decay; or, in other words, the general laws of matter, which had previously been suspended by the superior powers of life, once more come into operation, and give rise to definite chemical and physical changes. When the dead or decaying tissues communicate freely with the atmosphere, as in the different forms of gangrene, we at once recognise various well-known physico-chemical changes as the ordinary effects of the general laws of matter acting on animal substances subjected to certain conditions. But in the case of tissues not exposed to the air, comprising the various internal organs of the body, other and more gradual changes result from a complete or partial deprivation of their vitality.

The most frequent of these changes are softening, contraction or diminished bulk, induration, fatty degeneration, and calcareous degeneration; all of which morbid conditions are directly or indirectly connected with the diminution or cessation of the vital process of nutrition in the affected structures. The defective nutrition inducing these changes may either occur directly, as from old age, *or an enfeebled or diseased condition of the organs of circulation*, or as the result of local injury or disease, impairing or destroying the inherent vitality of the degenerated tissues, or *it may be induced indirectly or as a secondary effect of previous local inflammation or congestion. For the nutrition of a part is necessarily dependent upon the proper circulation of the blood through its capillaries; whereas in inflammation and congestion, the motion of the blood through the nutrient vessels is always temporarily, and often permanently and extensively, obstructed.* In inflammation, moreover, not only does the blood stagnate in the capillaries, and tend to coagulate in them, but lymph is at the same time also effused into the interstitial cellular tissue, and there partially organised, to the still further detriment of the normal capillary circulation. And when, at a subsequent period, the momentum of the arterial blood in the part is reduced by the cessation of the inflammatory action, the new products formed by the effused lymph, being themselves imperfectly nourished, also undergo retrograde changes or degenerations not very dissimilar to those taking place in the adjacent original tissues.

From these various causes, therefore, the capillaries of organs which have once been the seat of inflammation are to a greater or less extent permanently closed, the circulation of blood through the part is proportionally impaired, and the nutrition of the affected structures which depends upon the efficiency of the local circulation is consequently so far diminished as to render their feeble remnant of vitality incapable of resisting the general chemico-physical laws of matter.

Of the various changes enumerated:

Softening, or liquefaction, is simply the conversion of the tissues of an organ into a pulpy semi-fluid mass, the result of maceration, and is perfectly analogous to soft gangrene, the only difference being the absence of putrefaction, which is a chemical process requiring the presence of atmospheric air.

Contraction, or diminished bulk, is produced

partly by the absorption of the more liquid portions of the devitalised tissues by the blood-vessels of the adjacent living structures, and partly also by a peculiar tendency of abnormal fibro-cellular tissue to undergo a continuous process of contraction, which may, however, to a certain extent, be itself a result of the above-mentioned cause of diminished bulk.

Induration admits of a very similar explanation; its pathology being very analogous to that of contraction, and itself a frequent concomitant of that morbid condition.

Fatty degeneration offers one of the most interesting examples which pathological science has yet revealed of the wonderful extent to which obscure and deep-seated morbid changes may result from simple physico-chemical laws, brought into operation by the diminished vitality of the tissues of the living body. For in all essential particulars it corresponds to the change into adipocere of muscle and other animal structures, occasionally noticed when bodies have been for a length of time exposed to certain physical conditions.

Calcareous degeneration is the most unintelligible of all these morbid changes; for here we have not only a re-arrangement of the chemical elements of the decayed structures, but there is an absolute excess of one or more elementary substance (calcium and phosphorus), the source of which is not very easily explained. And though the received laws of chemistry, and the cautious spirit of inductive philosophy, at present enforce the conclusion, that the excess of phosphate of lime is deposited by the blood-vessels of the adjacent living structures, there are, I must confess, to my mind, great difficulties in accepting as final that solution of the mystery.

I have been tempted thus cursorily to review the changes occurring in organs wholly or partially deprived of their vitality, from the circumstance of my having been engaged at intervals, during the last ten years, in researches bearing upon this subject, the results of which are in general accordance with the views now adopted by many of the most distinguished pathologists in this country and on the Continent; and notwithstanding the flood of light cast upon the origin and nature of many of the morbid changes in question by the laborious investigations of those able observers, I hope to be excused for adducing even a small amount of concurrent testimony, which, as regards one form of degeneration, would appear to carry the inquiry a step further.

In 1843, this Society did me the honour to publish, in its Transactions, an account of some experimental researches communicated through the kindness of Dr. Marshall Hall, and having for their object the investigation of the immediate or primary effects of obstructed circulation in the kidney. These experiments have since been repeated by Frerichs, and my results confirmed by his more extended observations. I have also since applied the principles thence deduced to the explanation of the pathology and therapeutics of the earlier stages of inflammation, in a series of papers published in the "London Medical Gazette." But a prolonged observation of the secondary changes exhibited by the organs whose vitality was thus impaired, always appeared to me necessary to complete the investigation; and though the researches of Simon, Johnson, Virchow, and others, may have anticipated some of my results, the enumeration of the various effects which I have observed to follow the artificial obstruction of the circulation through the kidney, may yet not be altogether useless or uninteresting.

1. In the majority of cases, after ligature of the renal vein, or renal artery and vein, the kidney becomes enveloped by a cyst, formed of the surrounding cellular tissue infiltrated with blood and lymph, which cyst is speedily organised and retains the kidney *in situ*, thus preventing any liquefied portions of the dead organ from escaping into the cavity of the peritoneum. In the interior of this cyst the kidney, deprived of vitality, and no longer nourished by innumerable streams of blood incessantly permeating its structures, undergoes a process of *liquefaction*, or *softening*, which, commencing at the exterior, proceeds inwards until the more tenacious central portion is at length also reduced to a pulpy mass. After a period varying in different cases, the kidney is thus wholly converted into a puriform fluid enclosed within the cyst,—a pathological condition precisely analogous to that which we occasionally meet with in the human subject.

2. But, under certain circumstances, this protecting cyst is not formed, and I have accordingly, after complete obstruction of the renal artery and vein, found the kidney, at the end of twenty-four hours, reduced to a semi-liquid consistency, its pulpy mass

lying in contact with the intestines and other contents of the abdomen. The probable cause of this variation will hereafter be illustrated by an experiment.

3. In other observations I have found the kidney which had undergone congestion also unsurrounded by a cyst, but shrivelled, indurated, and paler than natural, thus exhibiting merely atrophy or *contraction* with *induration.*

4. In experiments where the kidney is found thus atrophied from obstructed circulation, as well as in those observations in which it undergoes slow liquefaction within a cyst, fat-globules can be detected in unusual quantity, showing a tendency to *fatty degeneration.*

5. I have lastly observed incipient *calcareous degeneration* to occur as the effect of the stoppage of the circulation in the kidney by ligature of the renal artery and vein. And as this is, as far as I know, a new fact in pathology, I may be allowed to relate the observation at length.

Exp. — On March 5th, 1853, the left renal vein and artery of a healthy young rabbit were closed by a tight ligature, which was allowed to remain; the cavity of the peritoneum was not opened, and the wound in the integuments being closed by sutures, very soon healed. On June 3rd, three months afterwards, the animal was in good condition; it had grown very much, and no abscess or other inconvenience had followed from the retention of the ligature. It was then killed. On opening the abdomen, the left kidney was seen of a pale yellow colour, and not half the size of the right, which was healthy, but somewhat enlarged.

The left kidney (the artery and vein of which were completely closed by the ligature) was enveloped by a cyst, on the surface of which some small vessels were perceptible. On dividing this cyst, a yellow pulpy matter was exposed, evidently formed by the disintegration of the cortical portion of the kidney, its central part being comparatively firm and natural. Near the pelvis of the gland, and at a point corresponding with the entrance of the vessels, was a loose calcareous ring, having in its centre a larger and a smaller circular aperture, its circumference being in contact with, and gradually thinning towards, the yellow pulpy matter. This latter, which was interposed between the internal surface of the cyst and the unliquefied portion of the kidney, when viewed by the microscope, consisted of granular matter, the particles of which varied in size, together with fat globules and crosses of altered hæmatosine.

On being allowed to dry, the pulpy matter became in parts semi-transparent, and opaque particles were distinctly seen to be imbedded in it. Being examined under a magnifying power, calcareous particles were perceived to be finely disseminated throughout the mass. A small piece of the dried pulpy matter was heated with liquor potassæ, and partially dissolved, emitting a peculiar odour. The sediment which remained was found, under the microscope, to consist of innumerable particles exhibiting different forms, some half-crystalline, others in the shape of spicula, rods, &c. Nitric acid being then added, these particles were dissolved. On heating a portion in the flame of a lamp, a copious white ash was left, which was not dissolved by acetic acid, but disappeared in nitric acid with very slight effervescence.

Such being some of the more frequent changes which impaired vitality produces in the internal organs of the body, it becomes a point of considerable interest, and great practical importance, to determine, as far as possible, the conditions which regulate the production of each of these particular effects. For by acting upon those conditions, we may sometimes hope to beneficially influence, or give a particular direction to, the change, or series of changes, occurring in different cases.

The investigation of this part of the subject has scarcely yet been commenced, but there are certain conditions which evidently affect the production of these pathological changes, among which may be enumerated the following:—

1. The chemical composition and physical structure of the tissues of the affected part, the relative proportion of liquid and solid matters which they contain, &c.

2. The physical and vital condition of the adjacent structures, their relative absorbing power, &c. I may illustrate this law by reference to the very different results which I obtained in experiments wherein the condition of the adjacent parts was the only essential variation. In the experiment already related at length, it was seen that the complete ob-

struction of the renal artery and vein was followed by the envelopment of the kidney in a cyst, the liquefaction of its external portion, and a diminution in its size as a whole; and that the central portion of the organ was comparatively firm and unchanged at the end of three months. In this case the peritoneum had not been opened, and there was no inflammation of it or of the intestines. In another experiment the renal vein alone was tied, and the animal allowed to live for three months, the peritoneum not being divided. At the end of that time the animal was quite healthy, there was no inflammation or suppuration in any part of the abdomen, and the ligature was merely surrounded by a little lymph. The kidney was healthy, its circulation being maintained unimpaired by a large lumbar vein which communicated with the vein of the kidney on the renal side of the ligature: whereas in another experiment in which the renal artery and vein were also obstructed by ligature, but in which the cavity of the peritoneum was accidentally opened, and the membrane exposed and inflamed, the whole substance of the kidney was found reduced to a pulpy state at the end of twenty-four hours after the application of the ligature. In this case, there was also no appearance of a cyst, the liquefied kidney being in contact with the inflamed peritoneum, from which a considerable quantity of serous fluid had been effused.

From various circumstances, I am, therefore, disposed to attach considerable importance to this point, believing that the condition of the surrounding structures often determines whether an organ whose vitality has been impaired by inflammation or otherwise, shall undergo a process of rapid and immediately destructive liquefaction, or shall be the seat of those more gradual and elaborate changes which do not in themselves so directly threaten life.

3. The temperature to which the affected tissues may be exposed.

4. The presence or absence of an investing cyst.

5. The presence or absence of atmospheric air.

6. The general vital condition of the body at the time, as modified by the quality of the blood, age, &c.

The imperfection of our knowledge on these and many other cognate questions, certainly indicates the necessity for continued researches into this important department of pathology; and if the present communication shall be found in any degree to encourage or facilitate farther inquiries, my object in thus troubling the Society will be fully answered.

ON

THE PECULIARITIES OF THE CEREBRAL CIRCULATION,

AND THEIR CONNECTION WITH

THE PHENOMENA OF EPILEPSY AND APOPLEXY.

[The greater part of this paper is taken from an unpublished work "On the Prevention and Treatment of Mental and Nervous Disorders."]

In addition to the functional disorders of the brain induced by inflammation and irritative debility, that organ is observed to be liable to a class of affections peculiar to itself, and usually described under the vague terms apoplexy and epilepsy.

Without previous symptoms further than those indicative of some irregularity in the flow of blood to and from the brain, the functions of the latter are suddenly suspended, and the patient sinks into a state of utter unconsciousness, accompanied either by the general loss of motor power, or by convulsions. After continuing in this condition for a certain length of time, the patient in epilepsy generally, in apoplexy often, recovers consciousness and voluntary motion, and may enjoy tolerable health until another attack occurs. Sometimes the person thus affected dies during the seizure, and on post-mortem examination there may be found some extravasation of blood or effusion of serum within the cranium; or a turgid condition of some of the cerebral vessels may exist; or, lastly, no morbid appearance whatever may be perceptible in the brain or other nervous structures. From the paroxysmal nature of the attacks, and from the occasional absence of all morbid appearances in the affected organ, it has been concluded that these diseases do not essentially depend upon structural lesion or change in the brain; while the premonitory and accompanying symptoms point to disorder of the cerebral circulation as at least a frequent coincidence in these singular maladies. Pathologists have therefore naturally been led to inquire, whether the arrangement of the brain and its blood-vessels presents any anatomical or physical peculiarities, and if so, whether those peculiarities are at all instrumental in producing, or are capable of rendering intelligible the occurrence of, the extraordinary disorders now under consideration.

Anatomy shows that the brain is differently circumstanced from other internal organs by being placed within a bony case which it completely fills, and by its venous blood being collected in large and strong intra-cranial reservoirs, prior to its discharge into the veins communicating with the heart. But while all pathologists agree in supposing these conditions, and particularly the former, to exercise a considerable influence upon the cerebral circulation, they are by no means agreed as to the mode in which its peculiarities operate. Some, reasoning upon the inelasticity of liquids, and fortified by the experiments of the late Dr. Kellie of Leith, have contended that the quantity of blood contained within the cranium is invariable; inasmuch as the brain, with its membranes and vessels, occupies the whole interior of a rigid globe, which, by the atmospheric pressure, is kept constantly filled. Others, disputing the accuracy both of Dr. Kellie's experiments and reasoning, and relying upon the congested appearance of the brain not unfrequently met with, and upon the evident expansion of that organ accompanying the ventricular contraction and the act of expiration (as seen after the operation of trephining), conclude that the quantity of blood in the cerebral vessels may be increased, and by its accumulation give rise to morbid phenomena. The latter view has recently been very ably supported by Dr. George Burrows, of London, while the arguments in favour of the Edinburgh doctrine, countenanced by Munro, Kellie, and Abercrombie, have been urged with equal force and clearness by the lamented Dr. John Reid, who was, however, careful to substitute the word "fluid" for "blood."* I must confess that the discussion of this question, up to the present time, seems to me scarcely to have embraced the point most immediately connected with cerebral pathology, and I feel the more at liberty to give utter-

* This doctrine has also received the able advocacy of Dr. Watson in his published Lectures; and by no pathologist has the whole question been more philosophically studied, or more effectually reconciled with the results of actual experience.

ance to this opinion, as I can agree, to a certain extent, with the views advocated on either side. The Edinburgh pathologists have, I think, satisfactorily proved that the variations in the absolute quantity of blood contained within the cerebral vessels as a whole are very limited, and that the brain, consequently, does not present the extreme and rapid sanguineous accumulations which we observe in other organs of the body. And I can, at the same time, equally agree with Dr. Burrows, that the *tendency to* such an accumulation of blood within the cranium may produce pressure upon the brain and its morbid consequences. The peculiar physical conditions affecting the brain, however, not only confine within narrow limits changes in the quantity of blood present in that organ, but, if I mistake not, they also exercise a still more important influence upon *the motion of the blood contained in its capillaries, and through it, upon the cerebral functions.*

I have previously alluded to the physiological law regulating the action of the nervous structures generally, and stated that the incessant motion of the blood through the capillaries of the brain is essential to the performance of its functions. Whenever, therefore, from any cause, external or internal, that capillary circulation is arrested, the functions of the brain immediately cease. If, then, it can be shown that, during an augmented flow of blood to, or its impeded return from, the brain, the physical conditions under which that organ is placed tend to arrest and obstruct the free passage of the blood through its capillaries, an explanation will, I conceive, be afforded of that sudden suspension of the cerebral functions which forms the most striking phenomenon in epileptic and apoplectic seizures. The brain, as we have seen, is contained in a rigid bony case, which it completely fills: it is, during life, of a semi-fluid consistence, and therefore capable of transmitting pressure equally in all directions. In its substance, and on its surface, are innumerable minute vessels, the coats of which are extremely thin; and through those vessels, in the healthy state of the organ, streams of blood constantly flow with considerable velocity; at its base are situated the large cerebral arteries, and along its upper and posterior portion are placed the strong and capacious sinuses communicating with the jugular veins. We observe that other internal organs, such as the liver and kidney, are liable to rapid enlargement as the result of an accumulation of blood in their vessels, originating either in an increased influx through the arteries, or a diminished efflux through the veins. And it is certain, from the observation of symptoms frequently present, as well as from the study of the anatomical, physiological, and pathological peculiarities and relations of the brain, that the arterial and venous tubes subservient to the motion of the blood through its minute vessels, are also subject to similar irregularities in their rate of discharge. What effect, then, will a suddenly-induced disproportion between the rates of influx and efflux of blood to and from the interior of the cranium, exercise upon the motion of that fluid in the minute vessels of the brain?

By a simple hydraulic experiment it can be proved that when the discharge from a tube is diminished by a comparatively slight obstruction, the lateral or distending pressure of the liquid situated behind the seat of obstruction rapidly approximates to and nearly equals the whole propelling force acting upon that liquid.* And when studying the phenomena of disordered circulation in the kidney, I obtained abundant evidence of the operation of this physical law in the hydraulic apparatus of the living body. For on artificially disturbing the natural proportion between the rate of supply of blood through the renal artery and its rate of discharge through the renal vein, the lateral or distending pressure of the intervening liquid was so great, that the organ contained an additional quantity of blood, equal, in some instances, to twice its original weight. The *enlargement* of the kidney in these experiments was, of course, very great.*

In congestion of the liver we also observe a rapid and considerable *enlargement* as the result of obstruction to the free flow of blood through the hepatic vessels. But when we proceed to study the operation of the same physical principle in the blood-vessels of the brain, we find its effects modified in a remarkable manner by the peculiar position of that organ. For however much the rate of efflux of blood through the jugular veins may be diminished, however much the rate of influx through the arteries may tend to increase, *the brain cannot materially enlarge;* it cannot burst the firm, unyielding walls which have grown

* Vide antè, pp. 75 and 154.

around it, and the general accumulation of blood in its vessels is thus mechanically prevented. The hydraulic law is, nevertheless, in full operation within the cranium. The venous sinuses will have a tendency to enlarge, the arterial columns will still endeavour to force their way into the smaller vessels, and the pressure and counter-pressure of the arterial and venous blood will thus be in existence to the same extent, and tend to produce the same general enlargement of the organ as in the liver and kidneys. That enlargement being, however, as we have seen, a physical impossibility, the distending force or pressure (which in other organs produces hyperæmia or congestion) is here communicated laterally to the whole semi-fluid mass filling the cranium, and through it to the external surface of all the capillaries of the brain. But these being thus compressed and flattened by the very force which in health propels the blood through them, no longer convey fresh streams of vitalising liquid to the nervous tissues, and the functions of the latter accordingly cease. According to this view, then, the same distending force of the impeded columns of blood, which, in other parts, leads to vascular enlargement, and, through it, to an increase in the bulk of the organ, is, in the brain, communicated to the circumjacent pulpy mass, and thus causes an external pressure which the thin membranous coats of the capillaries are unable to resist. Sudden and extreme irregularities in the flow of blood to and from the brain are therefore capable of inducing the complete and simultaneous stoppage of the capillary circulation in that organ, and with it the cessation of the cerebral functions, acting in this respect precisely in the same manner as other physical causes producing cerebral compression.

The arguments in favour of this opinion may be thus concisely enumerated:—

1. The incessant motion of the blood in the capillaries of the brain, is essential to the performance of its functions.

2. The brain cannot materially enlarge.

3. It is capable of transmitting pressure equally in all directions.

4. The natural proportion between the rates of supply and discharge of blood to and from the brain, is liable to be disturbed, and will then tend to produce a general accumulation in its vessels.

5. From the second proposition it follows that this general accumulation cannot take place in the brain.

6. The distending pressure of the impeded blood, which in other organs produces enlargement, is therefore, in the brain, diffused laterally and equally through the whole mass; it thus compresses and obstructs the capillaries, and, in arresting the ciren-lation through them, it also suspends the functions of the brain itself.

Having fully participated in the opinion expressed by a late eminent pathologist, that this subject required further investigation, I have been led to the conclusions now stated, with reference to the pathology of one class of cerebral disorders. And in leaving for the present the further consideration of irregularities in the *motion* of the blood as a source of disordered action of the brain, I cannot do better than quote the same writer's estimate of the importance of this study. "The circulation within the cranium" says Dr. John Reid, "possesses several peculiarities, which not only excite the attention of the anatomist, but are constantly referred to by the physiologist and pathologist, in their discussions upon the functions and diseases of the important organ there contained, viz. the encephalon. The derangements of the circulation within the cranium, are so often followed by such serious consequences, that it becomes an object of the highest practical importance to endeavour to ascertain the nature and cause of those derangements."

It will be seen that, according to this doctrine, the sudden compression of the brain (whether produced by an external injury, as by fracture and depression of the cranium, or by an internal disorder of the circulation) in giving rise to coma, acts by the stoppage of the blood's motion in the capillaries of the nervous structures. For the same pathological effect will always follow the same cause, so long as the surrounding conditions are unchanged.

Thus, the tendency to the accumulation of blood in the vessels of the brain, may arise from a suddenly increased influx of arterial blood, as from great excitement or exertion, or from a hypertrophied heart; or it may be induced by any circumstance impeding the return of blood from the lateral sinuses. And both in epilepsy and apoplexy, we observe in the predisposing and exciting causes a frequent proneness to the occurrence of one or both of those sources of disordered cerebral circulation.*

That the brain is in itself capable of considerable enlargement we see not only in the temporary elevation and expansion of the organ synchronously with respiration, in cases where it has been exposed by the operation of trephining, but also in the tension of the fontanelles in infants during paroxysms of anger or convulsions, and, in a still more striking degree, during the continuous and extreme augmentation of the head in chronic hydrocephalus.

While conversely in cases of death by hanging, it is found that though the eyes are almost forced out of the orbits, and the blood-vessels of the conjunctiva often give way under the pressure of the congestion, the integuments of the face and the scalp being at the same time inordinately swollen and engorged, the brain itself, which is equally exposed to the influence of the same obstructed circulation, remains comparatively unaffected in its appearance, and does not present anything like the intense degree of hyperæmia which might *à priori* have been expected.

* It has often occurred to me, that the careful examination of the state of the venous opening in the foramen lacerum posterius in fatal cases of epilepsy and apoplexy would materially assist in elucidating the pathology of those diseases. For as the greater part of the cerebral blood flows from the interior of the cranium through those small curved openings in the base of the skull, it is evident that any narrowing of them by thickening of the lining membrane, irregular ossification, &c., would create a constant liability to disordered circulation in the vessels of the brain.

ON THE

INFLUENCE EXERCISED IN HEALTH AND DISEASE UPON THE SENSORIAL FUNCTIONS OF THE CEREBRO-SPINAL NERVES

BY THE

STATE OF THE CIRCULATION IN THE ADJACENT BLOOD-VESSELS.

AMONG the conclusions most generally received respecting the physiology and pathology of the nervous system are the following: —

That the brain as the organ of the mind, can alone receive the impressions of sensation and originate those of volition.

That the gray matter of the brain is the active seat of its functions, and that its white fibrous portion is merely the conductor of those impressions to and from the former.

That the continuance of the functions of the brain is dependent on a constant and due supply of healthy arterial blood to the minute vessels of the organ.

That irregularities in the quantity, and deteriorations in the quality, of the blood transmitted to the brain will produce various disorders in its functions.

That the gray matter of the spinal cord is the great source of motific power; but that the excito-motory phenomena centring in it, may continue for some time after the total cessation of the circulation of the blood.

That impressions to and from the centres of sensorial and motor power, are conveyed along the cerebro spinal nerves, which are passive conductors of those impressions:

In reference to the special physiology of the cerebro-spinal nerves:

1. The researches of Sir Charles Bell have shown that the nerves proceeding from the spinal cord are anatomically and functionally compound, and that of the fibres constituting each nerve some are instruments of sensation, others of voluntary motion.

2. The demonstration of the special motor function of the spinal cord by Dr. Marshall Hall, renders it probable that purely excito-motory phenomena or involuntary muscular contractions are produced by impressions transmitted along nervous filaments intimately, if not exclusively, connected with the spinal cord.

3. The recent experimental investigations of Matteuci, moreover, tend to confirm previous ideas on the subject, in rendering it highly probable that the nervous power, which produces involuntary muscular contractions, is in its essential nature a physical force nearly allied to electricity.

All these researches merely assign to the cerebro-spinal nerves the power of passively conducting sensorial and motific impressions—as a wire conducts electricity; and they further assume, that as long as each nerve is structurally whole, and anatomically connected with the brain and spinal cord, it will continue to transmit impressions to and from these centres of nervous action. Now these conclusions are, doubtless, in a great measure, correct, as regards the transmission by the nervous fibres of motific or spinal impressions. For we find that in the bodies of animals recently killed, and after the circulation has entirely ceased, extensive spasmodic movements may be induced by irritating the spinal cord. But it appears to me, that the transmission by the same nerves of purely sensorial impressions, or those productive of sensation and voluntary motion, is accomplished under totally distinct conditions, and regulated by other and more essentially vital requirements than those above-mentioned. And I shall accordingly attempt to prove

1. *That a constant supply of arterial blood to the minute vessels of the cerebro-spinal nerves is required for the proper performance of their sensorial functions.*

2. *That local disorders of the circulation, affecting the blood-vessels of the nerves, are followed by corresponding irregularities in the transmission of the impressions of sensation and volition to and from the brain.*

And as corollaries from these laws, the following propositions may be deduced, viz.:

1. That the white or fibrous portion of the brain, which is identical in structure with the cerebro-spinal nerves, also, like them, requires for its nutrient vessels an incessant and normal supply of arterial blood in order to enable it to conduct impressions to and from the gray matter of the organ.

2. That the recognised necessity for that constant maintenance of the cerebral circulation, as a condition indispensable to the exercise of its mental functions, applies to the white as much as to the gray matter of the brain.

3. That the transmission of sensorial impressions along the cerebro-spinal nerves is a purely vital action, and, as such, quite distinct in its nature and in the laws regulating it, from the quasi-physical force producing excito-motory phenomena.

4. That, as regards their sensorial functions, the cerebro-spinal nerves are to be regarded as not only anatomically, but physiologically and pathologically, identical with the white or fibrous portion of the brain, and, consequently, as liable to the same physico-vital sources of disordered action as the brain itself.

In attempting to establish any law explanatory of the mysterious operations of the nervous system, it is above all things essential to discard pre-conceived ideas, and reason solely from *facts*. And, fortunately, the phenomena demonstrating the truth of the former of the two principal laws above stated, namely, the dependence of the sensorial functions of the nerves on the incessant circulation of the blood in the adjacent vessels, are so clear, direct, and adducible, as to render it wholly incontrovertible.

It has for many years been known that when a ligature is tightly applied to the abdominal aorta of any of the Mammalia, the hinder extremities are instantly paralysed. This circumstance was first noticed in experiments on animals; and, in the course of my investigations, I have frequently had occasion to observe the fact.*

In the few surgical cases where it has been deemed necessary to tie the abdominal aorta in the human subject, a similar effect has also been recorded. It was at first thought that the accidental retention within the ligature of some filaments of the aortic plexus of ganglionic nerves was the cause of the paralysis. But there can be no doubt that this explanation was fallacious, and that the paraplegia was simply the result of the cessation of the blood's motion in the minute vessels of the nerves of the affected limbs. For, as detailed in the experiments above referred to, and which are the more reliable as they were undertaken with another object, I have invariably found the connection between the stoppage of the circulation in the part and the production of the paralysis to be uniform and instant. On simply compressing the aorta with a forceps, the limbs receiving their supply of blood from it were at once deprived of sensation and voluntary motion. On allowing the blood again to flow into the femoral arteries, the animal within a few seconds regained the power of moving the hinder extremities, and "suddenly sprung up with a bound." In fact, the cessation and restoration of the sensorial functions of the nerves of the hinder extremities were, in these experiments, seen to be as clearly dependent on the presence or absence of the streams of arterial blood in the vessels of the part, as the action of a fountain

* Vide antè, Experiments on the Kidney, pp. 47, 48.

is on the influx of the liquid causing the jet. It should also be remembered that the nerves of the part were untouched and uninjured, and that their continuity with the spinal cord and brain was also perfect. The most evident and simple is, consequently, the only intelligible means of explaining the phenomenon.

The second, or pathological law, naturally follows the establishment of the physiological principle now stated. For, since the sensorial functions of the cerebro-spinal nerves, like those of the brain itself, are dependent on the normal maintenance of the local circulation, it is but in accordance with the general laws of disordered nervous action that an excessive or defective supply of arterial blood to the vessels of the part should produce corresponding variations in the intensity and activity of the functions arising from the circulation. Hence, an excessive supply of arterial blood produces the morbid sensitiveness and pain which we so often observe to accompany inflammation and determination of blood. And the influence of the opposite condition in diminishing nervous sensibility and the power of voluntary motion, is witnessed in the partial paralysis temporarily following the ligature of the secondary arteries, in the stagnating influence of extreme cold on the superficial capillary circulation and its consequent *benumbing* effect on the adjacent nerves; as well as the sluggish movements, the diminished sensibility, and the frequent tendency to local and functional paralysis of the various forms of anæmia.

From their possession of vital endowments equal

to those of the white matter of the brain, it would also appear probable that the nerves, like it, are capable of being affected in their higher functions by changes in the quality of the blood supplied to them, and of being variously acted on by medicinal substances locally applied. And there is every reason to believe such to be the case.

The further application of these principles to the prevention and treatment of nervous disorders, may be reserved for another opportunity, as it is not comprised within the leading object of the present work. But even the few remarks made may, perhaps, suffice to show how much we have yet to learn of the physiology and pathology of the least complicated nervous structures. They may also serve to illustrate the universality of the influence exercised in the living body by the simple, but wonderful, function, some of whose uses and disorders have, in the preceding pages, been briefly and imperfectly indicated.

THE END.

LONDON:
Printed by SPOTTISWOODE & Co.
New-street Square.

Spotted something that isn't quite right?

Let us know and we'll fix it for future reprints.
And as a thank you for your diligence, we'll
send you a free Sothis book of your choice.

publisher@sothis.press

This page intentionally left blank

Except of course for that line above. And this one.
And whilst we have your attention, perhaps you'd
like to follow us on Instagram @sothis.press. Go on.

Made in the USA
Monee, IL
08 November 2026

68113596R00173